MEDICO-LEGAL HAZARDS OF RUGBY UNION

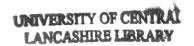
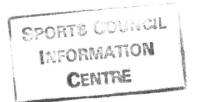

Medico-Legal Hazards of Rugby Union

EDITED BY

SIMON D.W. PAYNE

MB, BS, FRCS (Ed. and Eng.)
Assistant Secretary
The Medical Protection Society
London;
Department of General Surgery
Central Middlesex Hospital
London

CONSULTANT EDITORS

JOHN DAVIES

MRCS, LRCP, DPhysMed
Medical Director
Harley Street Sports Clinic
London

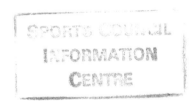

EDWARD GRAYSON

MA (Oxon)
of the Middle Temple and
of the South Eastern Circuit,
Barrister

FOREWORD BY

HRH THE PRINCESS ROYAL

PRODUCED WITH THE SUPPORT OF
THE WELSH RUGBY UNION

BLACKWELL SPECIAL PROJECTS·OXFORD

First published 1992

Printed and bound in
Great Britain by Hartnolls Ltd,
Bodmin, Cornwall

DISTRIBUTORS

Marston Book Services Ltd
PO Box 87
Oxford OX2 0DT
(*Orders:* Tel: 0865 791155
      Fax: 0865 791927
      Telex: 837515)

British Library
Cataloguing in Publication Data

Medico-legal hazards of rugby union.
  I. Payne, Simon D. W.
  617.1027

  ISBN 0-632-03183-2

To Eric, my father, who taught me
this noble game, and
Tom, the boy, who is learning

Contents

List of contributors

T. J. ANSTISS BM, MEd

Research Assistant, Charing Cross Hospital; Honorary Registrar, Ealing Health Authority, Ealing Hospital, Southall, Middlesex UB1 3EU; past international athlete

I. S. BENJAMIN BSc, MD, FRCS

Senior Lecturer, Royal Postgraduate Medical School; Honorary Consultant Surgeon, Hammersmith Hospital, Du Cane Road, London W12 0NS

M. BOTTOMLEY MB, ChB, DObstRCOG

Medical Officer, Bath University Medical Centre, Claverton Down, Bath BA2 7AY; Medical Officer to the British athletes team

J. DAVIES MRCP, LRCP, DPhysMed

Medical Director, Harley Street Sports Clinic, 110 Harley Street, London W1N 1AF; Consultant in Physical Medicine and Rehabilitation, The Devonshire Rehabilitation Hospital, Devonshire Street, London W1N 1RF; Honorary Physician to the Welsh Rugby Union; member of the International Rugby Board Medical Advisory Committee; Medical Officer to the British Lions

E. GRAYSON MA(Oxon)

Of the Middle Temple and of the South Eastern Circuit, Barrister, 4 Paper Buildings, Temple, London EC4 7EX

R. W. KENDRICK MB, FDS, FFD

Consultant Oral and Maxillofacial Surgeon, Northern Ireland Plastic and Maxillofacial Service, The Royal Victoria Hospital, Grosvenor Road, Belfast BT12 6BA; International Board and World Cup hockey referee

K. W. KENNEDY MB, BCh, DPhysMed

Consultant in Orthopaedic Medicine, 30 Harley Street, London W1N 1AB; past Irish international rugby player

B. KNIGHT MD(Wales), MRCP, FRCPath, DMJ(Path), Barrister

Professor of Forensic Pathology, Institute of Pathology, University of Wales College of Medicine, Cardiff Royal Infirmary, Newport Road, Cardiff CF2 1FZ

C. LOVEDAY MB, BS, MIBiol, PhD

Lecturer in Virology, Department of Virology, University College Hospital, London

D. A. D. MACLEOD MB, ChB, FRCS(Ed.)
*Consultant Surgeon, Lothian Health Board, West Lothian Unit, St John's Hospital
at Howden, Howden Road, West Livingstone, West Lothian EH54 6PP, Honorary
Medical Adviser to the Scottish Rugby Union*

K. MURPHY MCSP, DipPE
*Honorary Physiotherapist, The Commonwealth and Olympic Games, 1984, 1988;
British Lions, 1983, 1985; English Rugby Football Union since 1986; Chief of
Physiotherapy, BUPA Hospital, Whalley Range, Manchester*

S. D. W. PAYNE MB, BS, FRCS (Ed. and Eng.)
Assistant Secretary, The Medical Protection Society, 50 Hallam Street, London W1

J. G. P. WILLIAMS MD, MSc, FRCS, FRCP
*Consultant in Rehabilitation Medicine, Wexham Park Hospital, Slough, Berkshire
SO2 4HL; Medical Adviser to the Squash Rackets Association*

BUCKINGHAM PALACE

FOREWORD - HRH THE PRINCESS ROYAL

Organised sport forms an important part of the heritage of the people of the United Kingdom. Many of the games that are now enjoyed throughout the world have their origins in these isles, and the development of their rules of play and codes of conduct owe much to British influence in standards of civilisation and fair play. The United Kingdom is still in a position to influence those standards and this book could be a major factor in respect to medicine, sport and the law.

It is extremely important for the continued integrity of our society that the diverse activities enjoyed by so many, both as spectators and as participants, are seen to attempt to maintain a high reputation in terms of safety and standards of conduct. Unfortunately, in the same way that sport can be effective both in promoting health and causing injury, ever increasing standards of competitiveness and of professionalism, can likewise bring about progressively higher levels of excellence in conjunction with dubious standards of conduct. Our athletes continue to break world records but some will stoop to base levels and unfair methods in the attempt. The so called "professional foul" is now unfortunately only too well known in the context of competitive sport.

Sport can prevent its own destruction by appropriate action from its respective governing bodies. They will, however, need all the help they can muster and consequently it may be timely to enlist the assistance that medicine and the law may offer. It could also be argued that medicine and the law have already been enlisted - unfortunately for some of the wrong reasons - to research and prescribe undetectable drugs and arguments to avoid the rules of sport. The general conduct of sport at all levels will not improve if doctors and lawyers drive "four in hands" (coach and horses) through the spirit of the law.

However, when medical knowledge and research into the mechanism of injury is combined with relevant legal considerations, the results could offer sports legislators an excellent basis for sound reform of their rules with a view to increasing safety and eliminating undesirable practices.

The authors of this pioneering work have provided a much needed benchmark which may materially assist those involved in the assault on the problems which beset modern sport.

This book outlines the common medical and legal problems, and discusses some of the moral issues with which doctors attending sports men and women may be faced. By describing how these situations should be handled for the benefit and safety of sports men and women, this work has made a significant contribution to sports medical literature.

Preface

The success of *Medicine, Sport and the Law* in becoming a standard text of practical and authentic advice for doctors involved in sports medicine has stimulated the production of *Medico-Legal Hazards of Rugby Union* as an updated, streamlined and dedicated development structured specifically for the interest of team doctors in rugby union football.

Like its parent work, this volume seeks to explore legal, ethical and professional problems of relevance to the sports doctor in rugby football and is uniquely orientated to consider the particular clinical and medico-legal pitfalls that are associated with this game.

Although rugby union football endeavours to maintain its amateur status, standards of fitness, strength and performance spiral ever upwards producing an increasing capacity for injury. Both ordinary and elite participants will look to medicine to assist in their preparation, enhance their performances and treat their ills. A significant legal liability exists for doctors who attend such 'patients' in ignorance of their needs and it is vitally important to remember that neither the amateur status of the game nor the honorary nature of the doctors' attendance will provide immunity from litigation in professional negligence if inadequate or inappropriate standards of care have been applied.

Sports medicine is now established as a speciality in its own right, and rugby medicine is emerging as an important and legitimate subspecialism. Thanks to the enthusiasm and vision of my co-editor, Dr John Davies, and a number of leading figures in world rugby medicine, the first international conference on rugby medicine was held in Bermuda in November 1990. This provided the forum for an extensive and healthy exchange of information and ideas relating to the practice of medicine applied to rugby football. The proceedings of this conference, shortly to be published,* dovetail perfectly with the contents of this volume and together they form an important basis for on-going worldwide debate amongst the medical personnel who provide and are responsible for organisation of existing medical services in the context of rugby football. In considering how these services may be

---

Rugby Medicine (1991), the proceedings of the first international conference on rugby medicine, Bermuda, November 1990, edited by T. Gibson & J. Davies, Blackwell Scientific Publications, Oxford.

improved, it is important to remember that attention to the 'hands-on' service provided by skilled professionals to the 3.5 million people who play the game worldwide, is but the first line of approach. Alterations to the playing rules following conclusions reached as a result of research into sports medicine have already occurred and have helped to effect demonstrable reductions in casualties in the number of important contact sports. The role of the doctor in this regard must be to explain and maintain the pressure of medical evidence presented to the governing bodies in order that continuing beneficial amendments to the laws of the game are made. Continuing progress may be achieved only through the stimulation of further original medical research into all aspects of the game, so that patterns of injury may be identified and appropriate action instituted to minimise harm. Such research, properly conducted, critically appraised and scientifically presented may be harnessed through the broad scope of medical understanding for the benefit of players, administrators, spectators and the game itself.

SIMON PAYNE
London
July 1991

Acknowledgements

Many of the acknowledgements expressed in *Medicine, Sport and the Law* apply equally to this work as much of the basic material is the same. Significant additions, however, have been included as well as a number of amendments to update existing material, and the Editor is most grateful to the various contributors for their commendable punctuality within a tight schedule. It is hoped that this work will be of interest to International Rugby Unions, as the bodies ultimately responsible for instituting medical services to rugby activities within their jurisdiction. In this regard, Dr Roger Vanderfield, Chairman of the International Rugby Football Board, has shown particular enthusiasm for this project and the Editor is most grateful to him and his Committee for this support.

The majority of secretarial assistance necessary for production of the amended and additional material was provided by Miss Janice Thomson with the help of Miss Frances Azkue-Bright and Mrs Sue Brown who frequently provided both moral and actual support.

Mr Julian Grover has been most supportive throughout the complex gestation of this production and my thanks are due to him and his production team for their considerable understanding and co-operation in the face of impossible production schedules.

Finally, on the home front, Jet the dog remains serenely unperturbed, whilst Ailsa and Thomas continue to maintain the Editor's perspective and humility for which many thanks.

Medico-legal hazards in rugby football 1

SIMON D. W. PAYNE

'The Law marches with Medicine, but in the rear and limping a little'
L. J. Windeyer, *Mount Isa Mines Ltd* v. *Pusey* [1970], 125 CLR 383.

The Sports physician may be surprised to find that the application of law has an important role in sports medicine. Furthermore the normative medical values of physicians who provide their services to sportsmen and women, when combined with principles of law and ethics can, by synthesis of these two elements, produce a third element which may be characterised as an exercise in preventive medicine. It is important that doctors understand their responsibilities in both civil and criminal matters, and are also sensitive to the ethical pitfalls that exist for the unwary (Table 1). With regard to pitfalls of litigation the tort of negligence which traditionally has been perceived as having no application in sports medicine has produced a number of important reported cases where doctors providing their services to sportsmen and women have been found legally liable (q.v.). Furthermore, the issue may be complicated by the fact that the doctor–patient relationship can be significantly altered in sports medicine. Most doctors who provide their services in sports medicine do so on an honorary basis. Although there are a small number of dedicated sports physicians, in practice most are derived from the ranks of general practitioners or orthopaedic surgeons. In considering the doctor–patient relationship with respect to sports medicine it is helpful to consider first the types of relationship that can potentially exist. There are at least four types (Fig. 1.1). The first and most commonly encountered is described as the 'therapeutic relationship'. Here the doctor acts only in the best medical interests of his patient and exercises the fundamental principles of medical philosophy and practice for the benefit of his patient: to save life, promote healing and alleviate suffering. The application of these principles may be characterised as an exhibition of beneficence. Arising from the therapeutic doctor–patient

Material from this chapter taken from *Rugby Medicine* (1991), edited by T. Gibson & J. Davies, Blackwell Scientific Publications, Oxford.

relationship there are implications in issues of consent and confidentiality. In a therapeutic relationship the doctor is prohibited by his ethical code from disclosing secrets he learns about the patient unless the patient's consent is forthcoming. In other types of doctor–patient relationship there may be a responsibility to a third party, for example in the case of a medical examination for insurance purposes. Here the doctor will pass on to the insurance company information which, under normal circumstances, is secret and which the patient generally may not wish others to know. The doctor's position in this ethical matter is protected by virtue of the fact that the doctor always has (or should have) the patient's express consent to pass on that information. Similarly, doctors who work in various capacities for the State are called on from time to time to perform acts which cannot be construed as being beneficial to the patient. In the days of capital punishment, a prison doctor would be present to confirm death at judicial hanging; a function which cannot in any way be described as being in the patient's interest. Furthermore, in industry and other non-clinical branches of the health service doctors may provide information to other parties which in normal situations the patient may not wish them to do. A further example of modified doctor–patient relationship is seen in isolated communities, for example aboard ship and on expeditions to remote parts. The beneficence that a doctor would normally show towards an individual patient has to be taken in context with the viability of the expedition itself when the welfare of the party as a whole may conflict with the interests of an individual. Here the principles that would normally apply to save life, promote healing and alleviate suffering might not be expressed on a one to one basis as they would be in a normal therapeutic relationship.

Table 1.1
Responsibilities of the doctor in criminal and civil matters and ethical considerations.

Code	Purpose	Sanction
Criminal law	Protection of Society against undesirable activities	Fine or prison
Civil law	Protection of Society against poor standards (competence)	'Damages' paid in compensation
Ethical considerations	Maintenance of professional integrity (conduct)	Deregistration (GMC)

In research, on a philosophical level, no direct benefit will necessarily accrue to the individual patient as a direct result of the trial or experiment undertaken, other than through the benefit to society in general that may obtain through the advance in medical knowledge produced.

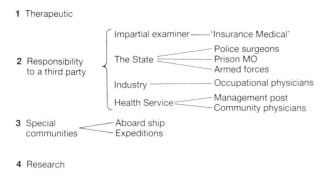

Fig. 1.1 Types of doctor–patient relationship.

As a separate parameter in the doctor–patient relationship, one should consider the varieties of attitude which the patient may exhibit with respect to autonomy. It is possible for the relationship at one extreme to be completely paternalistic and at the other for the control with regard to treatment and investigation to be devolved to the patient (Fig. 1.2). In British medicine a somewhat paternalistic attitude tends to be seen. Broadly speaking, patients seem happy to abdicate responsibility for medical decision-making to their doctor, perhaps because they do not particularly want to know the details of their investigation and treatment. This attitude, which tends to be more prevalent in older generations of patients, does, however, place upon the doctor a greater responsibility with regard to the standard of care he or she provides and should also cause the doctor to adopt a more cautious approach to investigation and treatment in the best interests of the patient.

This traditional approach should be contrasted with an alternative attitude which is emerging in which the patient demands greater autonomy over the medical decision-making process that takes place, producing a subtle change in the doctor–patient dynamic in which the patient defines an expectation with regard to the standard of care to be delivered in terms of 'rights to a level of quality'. This may be viewed as the counterpart of the duty of care of the doctor which is a more

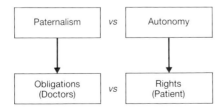

Fig. 1.2 Attitudes within doctor–patient relationships.

prominent feature within the framework civil law coloured by paternalistic attitudes. In consideration of attitudes with respect to delivery of health care the autonomous and paternalistic approaches may be thought of as being at opposite ends of the same spectrum. It seems probable that in a population of younger individuals, where sporting activity may be more prevalent, patients are more likely to wish to exert greater control over their own destiny in the investigation and treatment of conditions from which they suffer. Such a desire for greater autonomy may have its expression in a requirement for more detailed information about the investigation or treatment which the doctor is planning to provide.

The sports physician is therefore likely to be confronted relatively frequently with patients who demand greater autonomy with regard to treatment decisions and furthermore is quite likely to be providing a service where he may have a responsibility to a third party, such as a governing body or team management. It is likely that there will not be a strict therapeutic relationship between the doctor and the patient but that the relationship would be more akin to the type of doctor–patient interaction seen in occupational medicine. This is important because there are significant practical implications associated with the different types of doctor–patient relationship that may be seen. Normally, in a therapeutic relationship, there would be free and frank exchange of clinical information, possibly including details of a personal nature, between the patient's GP and any specialist to whom the patient was referred, where both practitioners are acting in a therapeutic sense. Generally there would be no need to obtain the patient's consent for such information to be transferred (although the patient's wish to prohibit such an exchange should usually be respected). Contrast this with the situation where the doctor has a responsibility to a third party, such as a 'company doctor' where the interests of the company have to be taken into account alongside those of the patient. Here the patient's express consent for disclosure is required. When a specialist considers the initiation of treatment for a patient, the GP's consent is not required where the relationship is of a therapeutic type, but consent from the GP should be sought before initiating treatment if the patient is seeing a doctor who is fulfilling the role of an occupational physician. Again this is because the function of the occupational physician is to provide advice to the organisation for which he or she works. This may involve determining a patient's fitness to work and whether or not any restrictions on the patient should be placed.

Assuming therefore that the sports physician sometimes functions in circumstances where he may not bear a normal therapeutic relationship with the patient and furthermore that he may be involved with patients who seek to exert greater autonomy over their destiny, consider the position of the team doctor who is approached by team management for medical information about a player which may affect team selection, where that player has asked specifically for that information to remain confidential. Clearly the doctor has an ethical dilemma, for to breach confidence by fully informing management of the complete nature of the player's condition could, on a theoretical basis at least, lead to censure from the doctors' disciplinary body (the General Medical Council) whereas to fail to disclose could possibly lead to economic loss arising from the poor performance of a key player for which the club could hold the doctor responsible if the facts became known. This potential problem could be eased if the relationship between the doctor and team management were to become more formalised. The doctor and his patient would then be more clearly aware of the nature of the relationship that existed between them, and commercial embarrassment between the doctor and the club would be avoided.

A definition of sport is difficult to find. The *Concise Oxford Dictionary* indicates that it is an activity in which enjoyment is an integral part. One of the best definitions has been coined by UNESCO: 'a physical activity which has the character of play and involves a struggle with oneself or with others in a confrontation of natural elements'. This is nevertheless an incomplete picture. Sport certainly involves exertion which is usually physical, although an intellectual game such as chess may be considered by many to be sport in which case the definition of 'exertion' ought perhaps to be widened to include physical or mental activity. Exertion nevertheless must be an integral part of the definition of sport in the same way that competition is also an element. A further factor which it is important to acknowledge is that there must be an acceptance of a framework of rules. Such rules exist on playing, organisation and national levels (Table 1.2). The regulations governing the shape of the pitch, the size of the ball, the number of players per team and the rules of play, both facilitative and restrictive, are all examples of playing rules. The administrative rules concerning the way in which the game is organised and set up within a given union are also well known. Many do not realise, however, that activities seen within the game, involving players, advisers and professionals, are also subject to national rules through legislation and the common law. Criminal law records a number of cases in which violent foul play has been a feature (Table 1.3). In each case a clear breach of playing and administrative rules has occurred which unfortunately were not dealt with effectively at these levels. The resulting unresolved grievances have therefore produced prosecutions for criminal assault, resulting in conviction in a number of cases, some with custodial sentences. In civil law the high water mark of litigation

Table 1.2 Rules of sport.	*Playing rules* Descriptive/facilitative Restrictive/penal
	Administrative rules Organisational Maintenance of standards and safety Disciplinary
	National rules Civil law Criminal law

Table 1.3 Criminal law in sport. *R.* v. *Bishop* [1986], *The Times*, 12 October.	1985: punched opponent in club match — concussion
	Playing rules Not seen by referee
	Administrative rules Ignored by club officials

	National 'rules'
	Prosecution for criminal assault
	   conviction
	     1 month imprisonment (reduced to suspended sentence by C/A)

between players on the pitch occurred in *Condon* v. *Basi* (Table 1.4). Here, during an amateur soccer match, a tackle in which a leg fracture was sustained was considered to be so gross a foul tackle by those who witnessed it that a successful suit in negligence and trespass was brought and damages of some £4000 were paid.

Doctors who have traditionally thought themselves immune from civil litigation when providing their services in a sports context may wish to consider the salutory case of *Robitaille* v. *The Vancouver Ice Hockey Company Ltd* (Table 1.5). Mike Robitaille was a professional ice hockey player whose repeated complaints of injury were ignored by the club doctor. He sustained damage which curtailed his playing career and the doctor and the club were found negligent. The club was adjudged vicariously liable for the doctor's

Table 1.4 Civil law in sport. *Condon* v. *Basi* [1985], 2 AER 453.	Foul tackle during amateur soccer match — broken leg
	Claim in negligence and trespass
	£4000 damages awarded (affirmed in C/A)

Table 1.5 Medical liability in sport. *Robitaille* v. *Vancouver Ice Hockey Club Ltd* [1981], 3 DRL 288.	Professional ice hockey player: repeated complaints of injury

	Club doctor (no contract) provides incomplete examination and no effective treatment
	   Neck damage not diagnosed
	   Playing career shortened

	Doctor and club found negligent (club vicariously liable)
	Award $175 000 for loss of professional hockey income $85 000 for future loss of other income $50 000 for pain, suffering and loss of amenity
	Total $310 000

negligence and this was perhaps fortunate for the doctor because otherwise he could have been made personally liable. An award of over $300 000 in damages was made in 1981, upheld on appeal. This result exemplifies how civil liability is an important issue for doctors providing their services to sports people and doctors so affected are usually personally liable.

Civil liability is a risk for all professional practice. A confusion may arise because the dictionary definition provides an English linguistic understanding of the word negligence which is significantly different from the legal definition. This is strictly defined as 'a breach of duty of care resulting in damage'. There are thus three elements: a duty of care between the doctor and his patient; a breach of that duty; and loss or damage. The law of negligence exists to provide compensation for loss which may include pain, suffering, loss of amenity and economic loss. The common law and its system of precedent will determine fairly consistently the monetary value which may be associated with pain, suffering and loss of amenity of various kinds. Economic loss, however, is very variable and depends on such things as earning capacity of the individual and the extent to which this has been compromised, and the number of productive years the individual could have expected to have enjoyed had these not been curtailed by the act of negligence. The professional responsibilities or the duty of care which the sports physician owes to his patient should be recognised wherever a sporting injury requires treatment, a breach of that duty alongside a reasonably foreseeable risk of injury creates a liability in negligence. The standard of care required is determined under English law by the case of *Bolam* v. *Friern Barnet Health Authority*, a landmark case in medical negligence. This is defined as the standard of 'the ordinary skilled man exercising and professing to have that special skill: a man need not possess the highest expert skill. It is sufficient if he exercises the ordinary skill of an ordinary competent man exercising that particular art'. Doctors providing services in sports medicine are therefore required to display the skill of the average sports physician. The fact that the average standard of such practitioners is increasing through education means that a doctor must achieve a level of competence which is significantly higher than that of even a few years ago. Litigation in medical practice generally is on the increase on both sides of the Atlantic. The Canadian Medical Protective Association's analysis of their legal action per 1000 members indicates an approximate 10-fold rise from 1960 to 1986. In the USA malpractice settlements are also increasing and by 1985 the average litigation settlement for medical malpractice had exceeded £1 million. There are a number of reasons for these massive numbers seen in North America, not least of which is the use of the contingency system. This means that the lawyer running the case is paid nothing if the case is lost but receives a substantial payment if the case is won, up to 50% in some incidences. It is, however, felt that this system provides a greater accessibility to the law for the general public, as contrasted with the system seen in the UK where one's legal fees to solicitors and barristers are payable whether the case is won or lost. A further important difference between the USA and UK systems is that in the USA malpractice cases are tried by jury, who also may determine the quantum of damages. In the UK similar cases are heard by a High Court judge sitting alone.

It is important to remember that for doctors who are touring abroad, medical services provided therein are subject to the local jurisdiction and a touring doctor could therefore be sued within these courts. It is essential therefore that any doctor accompanying a visiting team who contemplates undertaking any medical procedure of whatever description is adequately covered by insurance. This may be a particular problem for the USA and Canada where the UK protection organisations do not write business.

Doctors who associate themselves with sports medicine have a duty not only to treat patients who appear with injuries, but also to endeavour to reduce the incidence of injury by collecting and analysing information in order that patterns of damage may be identified.

The American Association of Neurologists has produced striking improvements in the nature and extent of injuries occurring to American professional football players following a study taking place between 1968 and 1973. This led to modifications of laws, equipment and coaching techniques and illustrates what can be done if the full force of medical evidence is presented to governing bodies in a way which cannot be ignored. Likewise the Medical Committee of the International Rugby Football Board (IRFB) have made certain recommendations with respect to playing and administrative rules which have brought about a reduction in certain injuries (Table 1.6).

Table 1.6 Preventive medicine in sport. Recommendations of the Medical Advisory Committee, 1978.

Elimination of high tackle

Scrummaging law changes
   reduce impact
   prevent collapse
   prevent scrum rotation

Maul v. ruck
   encourage players to stay on feet
   encourage quick release after tackle

Drugs/doping — no injectable analgesics

Player size (schools) — avoid mismatch

Mouthguards

Concussion — 3 week ban

The team doctor in rugby union football 2

K.W. KENNEDY

'A ruffians sport played by gentlemen'
Anon

Doctors who are considering providing services in the context of rugby football ideally should have a sound knowledge of traumatology and the kinesiology of the sport. Most importantly the doctor should have an affinity for the game and the people in it. It is helpful also if the doctor has good contacts within the profession in order to facilitate referral in cases where this is appropriate. Experience in rehabilitatory medicine or orthopaedics is invaluable and the ability to liaise concisely with physiotherapists is nowadays most important, so as to ensure the safe return of the player to his sport as quickly as possible. In rugby football the duties of a team doctor are mixed. On match days prior to the game the doctor will have liaised with the coach and manager to ensure that players are aware of, and ideally should have taken, an optimal pre-match diet. In the dressing-room the doctor will be expected to assist with strapping of joints where necessary. Often players will ask for a pain-killing injection prior to playing. This practice is to be avoided. Moreover, the request should not arise if the selectors and coach have agreed beforehand that an injured player should be rested until he is fully recovered. During the game, the doctor, although metaphorically 'in the background', should actually be in the forefront of availability, ready to help with any injury that occurs. The doctor should actually therefore be available somewhere near the touch-line, and not in the back of the grandstand or, worse still, in the committee bar!

The responsibility of the team doctor

The principles of preventive medicine should be high on the list of priorities when a team doctor is considering the list of his duties.

At the start of a season both the coach and the doctor must advise the players on many topics.

Training

Training involves consideration of the total musculoskeletal system and includes:
1 Mobility and flexibility training.
2 Breathing controls.

10

Chapter 2
The team doctor
in rugby union
football

3 Muscle training and building.
4 Co-ordination improvement.
5 Game skill techniques.

Kit

The pressures of commercialism cause some manufacturers of sports goods to pay a lot of attention to their logos and brand names and less to the quality of their product. Boots and track shoes are probably the most important item of equipment and should be carefully chosen. The current vogue for cutaway boots does much to increase the profit of the manufacturer (who uses less leather), but does little to protect the ankles of the players, thus increasing the possibility of ligament injury and long-term 'footballer's ankle', a type of degenerative joint disease.

Rugby players are notorious for failing to wash their training kit. This can lead to serious skin infections, interfering with the individual's availability for both work and competition.

Although initially viewed with suspicion, protective kit is now accepted by players and nowadays no player should neglect to wear appropriate protective wear. The gum-shield should be worn by all players who still possess teeth. Modified shoulder padding should be used by those players who have had recent or recurrent shoulder injuries. All forwards, and especially front-row players, should be encouraged to wear shin pads to prevent the common stud injuries to the slow-healing skin on the anterior aspect of the tibia. Protective knee and elbow braces are available but these should only be used after specialist opinion has been sought.

Diet and rest

Advice should be given to players on the need for proper sleep in the days before a major game. Changing the diet of the players is more difficult. It is advisable to eat sensibly before a big game but this must be coupled with timing of training. It is well known that a decreased glycogen storage and low blood-sugar levels impair the physical and mental performances of players and also increase their injury risk factor. Physiologically it takes about 36–48 hours to build up the glycogen stores by taking a diet high in carbohydrate content. Thus it is obvious that no hard training sessions should be held within 48 hours of a game or else the stores will be burnt up and none remain for the game. This often has been a reason for the lack-lustre performances of certain teams in the past. They have left their energy on the training ground due to poor management and have little to give in the big match.

11
*Chapter 2
The team doctor
in rugby union
football*

Psychology

Sport is littered with psychosomatic cripples and rugby is no exception. The team doctor must play a firm and sympathetic role in preparing the player for the sport. The sportsman or woman produces their best when top physical condition gels with the ideal psychological approach. The ability of a player to concentrate under extreme conditions is essential in sport. Too much or too little mental tension adversely affects concentration. In future seasons the doctor may be expected to help the player with this, and techniques such as biofeedback and meditation have been used with great success in golf and tennis.

Treatment of injuries

Effective sports medicine offers the injured player early assessment and prompt treatment. It is necessary to start evaluating the problem from the moment of the injury; if the accident is witnessed by the doctor who has a knowledge of the kinesiology of rugby, then establishing the diagnosis is made simpler. It is vital that after the injury the patient is not made worse by some well-intentioned but untrained person. It is all too easy for a simple fracture to be turned into a compound one, or for a fractured cervical vertebra without neurological problems to be converted by bad management into a neurological disaster. At all sports grounds where vigorous bodily contact sport takes place, suitable personnel and equipment should be available. These should include:

1 Trained personnel on duty, including doctor/physiotherapist.
2 Spinal stretcher and blankets.
3 Working telephone and list of emergency numbers.
4 Ice-packs.
5 First-aid kit, which should include:
  (a) Brooke airway;
  (b) tongue depressor;
  (c) suture kit;
  (d) slings;
  (e) splints;
  (f) disinfectant;
  (g) bandages and cotton wool;
  (h) analgesics;
  (i) disposable gloves.

In 1981 a survey was done of rugby clubs in Surrey and it was found that very few possessed these minimum requirements.*

*The responsibility for providing these items of equipment rests with the governing body of the home club. It would be prudent, however, for the team doctor to bring to the attention of the committee any perceived inadequacy in the first-aid equipment.

12

Chapter 2
The team doctor
in rugby union
football

When assessing an injured player it is helpful for the doctor to have some guidelines to assist in making the decision as to whether he should leave the field of play. It is important that all concerned — coach, captain and player — know that the doctor is making the decision to safeguard both the player and his team-mates. Sometimes players unwisely stay on the pitch following injury and in so doing put themselves and others at further risk. The following injuries should be viewed as absolute indications to retire from the field of play:

1   Major laceration.
2   Severe muscle or tendon tear.
3   Dislocation of a major joint.
4   Head injury.
5   Spinal injury.

Major laceration

If a wound is deep, and especially if vital structures such as arteries or nerves are exposed, or if joints are involved, then, even if the function of the part is normal, the player should be advised to leave the pitch. Routine cleansing, antibiotics and antitetanus treatment should be effected as well as suturing the wound, although it is likely that a wound of such severity would require formal exploration and debridement under regional or general anaesthetic, to check the integrity of vital structures and to ensure complete removal of all foreign material. Under normal circumstances this of course means referral to hospital.

Muscle or tendon injury

If the tear is sufficient to limit function, then the player is at risk of further damage. If the muscle injury is associated with haematoma, then prompt initial treatment with compression and elevation of the injured part is likely to prevent troublesome sequelae. Unfortunately, as it is the lower limbs that are commonly injured in rugby football, this form of therapy makes it necessary for the injured player to adopt a recumbent position with leg elevated above the level of the head. Too frequently, social pressures cause such players to abandon therapeutic measures after cursory treatment and they are often to be found standing in the club bar with their team-mates after the game. The resultant oedema, however, will significantly lengthen recovery time.

Dislocation

Major joint dislocation normally gives extreme pain and loss of function and the player usually has no wish to continue. Dislocation of the interphalyngeal joints can often be reduced by experi-

13
Chapter 2
The team doctor
in rugby union
football

enced personnel and the player allowed to continue, though neighbour strapping and a follow-up X-ray are essential. Major dislocations, especially when complicated by fracture, should be referred immediately to hospital for treatment. Shoulder dislocation can be reduced immediately if a significant delay in hospital attention would otherwise occur; care, however, should be taken to assess the patient for fracture of the humerus, which may cause damage to the axillary nerve as a complication of the dislocation. In cases of doubt, treatment should be delayed until X-ray examination has taken place.

Fracture

The signs of fracture are:
1 Deformity.
2 Abnormal mobility.
3 Crepitus heard and felt.
4 Local bone tenderness.
5 Loss of function.
In all cases of fracture the patient should be kept warm and moved as little as possible. The fracture should be splinted if possible before referring to the local hospital.

Head injuries

Any player who has had a loss of consciousness during play must take no further part in the game. This applies also to anyone who has suffered concussion. Concussion is a syndrome in which there is immediate impairment of neural function following a blow to the head. The player with the glazed look and rubbery legs is a danger to himself and others. Speed of reflex actions will become markedly reduced and he becomes prey to the 'sucker punch'.

In boxing now there is a statutory period of four weeks' enforced inactivity after a knock-out, and the same could be considered reasonable for all sports. Prior to playing again after head injury, the player should have a complete medical check-up.

Spinal injury

Amongst the most serious injuries in sport are the fracture, fracture–dislocation and dislocation of the cervical spine. These conditions are surgical emergencies and the risk of paraplegia is high if management is incorrect.

Horse-riding, rugby, rock-climbing and judo are the sports in which neck injuries are common. When faced with the problem of the player who falls awkwardly and stays down immobile, the doctor, the trainer and indeed anyone on the field of play should be aware of the physical signs which indicate serious injury to the cervical spine:

14
Chapter 2
The team doctor
in rugby union
football

1 Loss of function in the limbs.
2 Deformity of the neck.
3 Unconsciousness.
4 Complaint of parasthesia in limb(s).

In the presence of these findings extreme care must be taken. An incomplete cord lesion can be converted into a complete one by improper handling.

Initial treatment

The first task is to ensure that the airway is patent and that normal breathing is occurring. The mouth must be examined immediately to remove the mouth-guards, chewing-gum and other foreign bodies such as broken teeth, and to ensure that the tongue is not obstructing the airway. These emergency measures having been taken, the injured player should not be moved until someone trained in moving a suspected cervical spine injury case is present. The patient should be kept warm by covering with blankets or coats.

Intermediate treatment

The patient should be transferred on to a special spinal stretcher. It is essential that the transfer of the patient from the ground to the stretcher is properly supervised, the aim being to support adequately the patient's neck. Three helpers on each side help lift the patient on to the stretcher, working in unison under the command of the trained person. Once the patient's condition has been stabilised, he should be transferred to a hospital for investigation and treatment.

Other injuries requiring hospital treatment

Trauma to the eye, genitals or serious intra-abdominal injury usually produce a shocked patient who should be treated for the shock along standard lines and referred to hospital as appropriate.

High-risk situations

When an analysis is made of the mechanism of rugby injuries, certain factors stand out.

General

1 Mismatch. When opponents are roughly the same size and strength for their position, they are usually able to cope with the stresses of the game. When this is not the case, such as in schoolboys versus adults rugby matches, then the risks increase. This is especially pertinent to school rugby, where children should be matched by size and not age.

2 Incorrect equipment. No player should be allowed to take the field or to participate in opposed training in incorrect or inadequate kit, e.g. a forward using track shoes in a scrum instead of boots is 50% more at risk.

15

*Chapter 2
The team doctor
in rugby union
football*

3 Unfit or inexperienced. Not infrequently a veteran, who may be unfit, is asked at the last minute to play or practise against strong opposition. Once, on an Irish tour in Australia an assistant manager, who was a past international forward, packed down in the front row without boots against the test side to illustrate a point. He emerged from the top of the scrum with two broken ribs — a sorry sight and a very chastened man.

4 Horseplay or foul tactics. There are still, unfortunately, individuals playing rugby who appear to derive pleasure from injuring their opponents. It is the duty of club members and selection committees to weed these people out as they have no place in the game.

Specific

1 Mistackle. Probably one of the commonest causes of serious injury. Serious neck injuries can occur if the tackler's head collides with the opponent's hips or thigh. This usually occurs when the tackler closes his eyes and/or does not position his head correctly to the side or behind the thigh of the oncoming opponent. The best prevention of this type of injury is thorough coaching and practice of correct technique.

2 Short-arm tackle. This occurs when the opponent changes direction at the last minute and goes inside the tackler, who throws up his extended arm, usually hitting the opponent across the throat or face, causing a whiplash type injury to the neck. The short-arm tackle is illegal within the laws of the game.

3 The pile-up. This describes a situation where a loose scrum evolves as forwards dive into it to win the ball. Those at the bottom may be injured by the force of the in-charging players. The rules regarding this have been recently improved and referees are recommended to stop play early if a collapsed scrum situation develops either in loose play or from a set piece.

4 The set scrum. Serious neck injuries can occur in association with the set scrummage. The front-row players are primarily at risk. In the set scrum the danger times are:

(a) impact. When the scrums pack down and the front rows collide shoulder-to-shoulder. Faulty timing of one player may cause his head to collide against his opponent's head or shoulder with obvious risk of injury;

(b) collapsing scrum. When the scrum has settled after the impact of the two sets of forwards, it may collapse unintentionally or be collapsed deliberately. There are many ways a scrum can be made to

16

Chapter 2
The team doctor
in rugby union
football

collapse which are not in this brief. The most obvious is the prop forward pulling down his opponent. With experienced players this is not usually dangerous as most competent front-row players have practised how to fall. It is usually when there is a mismatch in physique or experience between opposing front rows that injuries occur. The most dangerous part of a collapse situation occurs when the second and back rows continue to push whilst the heads and necks of the front-row players are trapped against the ground. This can be prevented by the education of players and the prompt whistle of the referee;

(c) aerial serum. This is one of the most frightening and dangerous experiences for front-row players. It may happen when an entire front row is lifted off the ground by the superior technique of their opposition, whilst their own second row continue to push. The trapped players risk severe damage to their cervicothoracic spine, and any forward who has been in this situation speaks of his helplessness and fear. It is also the situation where 'sprung ribs' or fractures at the costochondral junction may occur.

Methods of reducing risks of injury

1   Players:
    (a) must be fit;
    (b) always wear correct equipment;
    (c) do not play out of position;
    (d) do not indulge in horseplay or foul play.
2   The coach:
    (a) does not select unfit players;
    (b) ensures that the skills of the game are learned and practised; this includes tackling, falling and scrummaging.
3   The referee:
    (a) must stop the play at once when a set scrum collapses;
    (b) must stop the play at once if a loose scrum becomes a fight or collapses;*
    (c) should punish severely (sending off, followed by club disciplinary action) repeated use of illegal techniques such as the short-arm tackle.
4   Administrators have a duty to keep the laws of the game under constant review with a view to improving safety for players and taking into account the evidence available from relevant research (see also Chapter 10).

---

* Intentional collapse of the scrum is of course illegal within the laws of the game. The difficulty for the referee arises in deciding which of the front rows were responsible for causing the collapse. The intricacies and tactics of front-row play are beyond the scope of this text. It seems clear, however, that the extremely serious form of injury resulting from this can be prevented most effectively by prompt action by the referee.

17
*Chapter 2
The team doctor
in rugby union
football*

Conclusions

It is important that the doctor who undertakes the task of the team medical officer in rugby football should understand, enjoy and respect the sport which he or she serves. Likewise he or she should command the respect of the players and administrators whom he or she advises, so that unwelcome counsel is not ignored when it matters, e.g. advice to leave the pitch following injury. As long as rugby union football remains amateur, the status of the club doctor will probably be honorary. He or she, like the coach, gives his or her time freely without tangible reward. The team doctor has an important role in rugby which can be enormously rewarding.

Recommendations

1 In England a restructuring of the game has seen the emergence of four divisional teams. It is suggested that centres of medical excellence should be set up for each of these where:

(a) injured players can be referred by club doctors and GPs to be seen by sports medicine specialists appointed by the Rugby Unions;

(b) a regular teaching commitment should be undertaken for team doctors, physiotherapists and first-aiders, etc.

2 The Rugby Football Union and other international unions give due attention to the issue of safety. It is suggested that, in addition to ongoing attention to the rules of the game, prescriptive requirements are made with respect to the adequacy and provision of first-aid personnel and equipment at the grounds of affiliated clubs.

3 It is suggested that any player who has received a serious injury (one that has necessitated him leaving the pitch) may only restart playing after he has had medical clearance to do so. The system employed in France could be adopted. Here all players of recognised clubs are issued with a 'licence' card. These record the personal disciplinary and injury record of each player. At the end of each season they are collected centrally for analysis and contribute greatly to a better understanding of the patterns of injury occurring within the game.

4 It is recommended that all players should be encouraged to take out adequate personal injury and disability insurance. In the United Kingdom affiliated clubs of the Rugby Football Union may take advantage of corporate and individual policies offered.

3 The team doctor in international rugby football

J. DAVIES

'A gentleman's sport played by ruffians'
Anon

As in all aspects of the profession, a doctor's prime function is advisory and nowhere is this more paramount than in the role of a medical officer to a national body, such as the Welsh Rugby Union (WRU). Besides advising on dope-testing, the role of the team doctor encompasses advice on vaccinations, medication and the general primary medical care of the squad.

The role of the team doctor

The medical needs of players in the national squad, whether at training sessions, at international weekends or on tour, are the responsibility of the team doctor. It is important to gain the players' confidence. The easiest way to do this is to involve oneself totally with the team's preparations, e.g. working closely with and assisting the physiotherapist in strapping techniques, and perhaps supervising the warm-up and pre-activity stretching exercises at training sessions. Familiarity, some people say, breeds contempt, but for rugby players, each with their own idiosyncrasies and superstitions, it is essential for them to have complete confidence in their team doctor, especially when playing conditions are adverse.

A prop forward, waking up on the morning of an international with a slightly wry neck following the previous day's scrummaging practice, or a wing threequarter, still troubled with a slight hamstring pull, must have the confidence to approach the doctor. In the case of the former, the author remembers a case where no approach was made to the doctor concerned and, as a result, the Wales scrummage had their worst performance in recent years. The prop eventually went off with cervical spasm, and Wales lost the match! As in any doctor–patient relationship, if there is a case for treatment, whether it be an infected ear, a swollen proximal-interphalangeal finger joint, a blister or just ligament or muscle problems, treatment must be instigated as early as possible. Drugs such as antibiotics or anti-inflammatory agents are occasionally supplied to players, or alternatively they may be advised after a training session, when indicated, to obtain a prescription or seek advice from their own general practitioners. Where physiotherapy is required, the patient's team physiotherapist will liaise with the physiotherapist of the player's own club.

During international matches, injuries do occur and players are occasionally substituted. One of the greatest concerns for the medical officer officiating in any collision/physical contact sport such as rugby is the occurrence of a serious spinal injury. The scoop stretcher has been designed with the spinal injury in mind and in order to produce the least possible chance of spinal damage. The ground staff should be trained to move a patient with suspected spinal injury: the player should be transferred to the stretcher by three on either side with the head being held in traction. At Wales National Stadium during international matches an ambulance is on standby, and there is a direct line available to the Cardiff Royal Infirmary for immediate admission if required. Other international rugby stadiums have similar equipment and emergency procedures available.

The team doctor must work very closely with the national team coach and his assistant, and also should liaise closely with the selectors, and must gain the confidence and respect of both parties. In the match situation the doctor can sometimes be of assistance to the coach and selectors by identifying subclinical injuries in players which may be apparent on close observation of their performance, e.g. a player favouring one leg. For each international, the doctor has to confirm that a player of his or her side is unable to continue the game, or that it would be inadvisable on medical grounds for that player to continue, before a substitution is allowed. Speed is of the essence in this situation, and occasionally before a player is substituted it has been known for the team doctor to advise the coach that a certain player has a problem, in order that the replacement can be adequately warmed up before going on to the pitch.

The laws of the game now state that treatment can be continued on the pitch whilst the game is in progress and this has certainly helped reduce the time for stoppages due to minor injuries. The team doctor is not allowed on to the pitch unless specifically signalled for by the referee. This may occur following a request by the trainer/physiotherapist who is already on the field, or the referee may make the decision himself if the injury obviously warrants a doctor's immediate attention.

The laws of the game at present state that no more than two players in each team may be replaced and a player who has been replaced may not resume playing in the match. In international matches, a player may be replaced only when, in the opinion of a medical practitioner, the player is so injured that he should not continue playing in the match.

If a referee is advised by a doctor or other medically trained person or if he for any other reason considers that a player is so injured that it would be harmful for him to continue playing, the referee shall require the player to leave the playing area.

The author recalls an incident in which a district club side which he was coaching was due to start a match against strong West Wales opposition without the benefit of their outside half, who had failed to turn up. The author was recruited to the team, but shortly after taking the field the missing player appeared on the touchline, having been delayed in traffic and hastily changed in his car on arrival. The delayed player signalled his wish to join the game but the author, although relieved, realised that such a substitution could not be automatic. A convenient minor injury occurred soon after this, and at the resulting stoppage in play the author declared himself unfit to continue. The referee, quite rightly at the time, informed the trainer and the author that no replacement would be allowed. The author duly informed the referee, to his total bewilderment and confusion, that he was a doctor, and limped off. The fly half ran on, but the matter did not end there. Two of the opponents' committee were unhappy and the author was followed to the changing-room. It was only the sight of a patellectomy scar which the author had fortunately acquired several years previously that appeased them, although not without a great deal of muttering and disbelief.

The law has subsequently been amended such that an injured player may be replaced:
1 at the advice of a medically trained person, or
2 if a medically trained person is not present, with the approval of the referee.

As physician to the WRU one's advice is sometimes sought on medical and medico-legal matters.

The medical advisory capacity also includes lecturing to coaching conferences at a national level on medical matters such as conditioning, diet, body composition, effects of training and also injuries and their treatment. The WRU has nine districts, comprising in total 200 clubs, and in recent years each district has received lectures (with representatives from each club in attendance) on the necessity for and organisation of medical cover and the treatment of rugby injuries.

In the weeks preceding overseas tours, advice is usually also sought on the need for vaccinations if indicated. Together with the tour physiotherapist, lists of essentials are made bearing in mind the countries to be visited.

Psychological pressure at international level

Psychological pressures on players associated with an approaching rugby international are intense (and more so when playing in Wales). There is no escape from the media, well-meaning friends, ticket-seekers and critics. This overwhelming exposure must and does have an effect on the participants, in particular on newcomers to the international arena.

The Welsh team, replacements, coach, selectors and team doctor meet the day before a home international and stay overnight, all the training and technical work-outs having been completed. If any last-minute medical problems arise, they are dealt with and the evening is spent relaxing, usually watching a film on video. The players retire around 11 p.m. Over the years very few players have asked for hypnotics to help them sleep and, on the rare occasions that it was necessary, they have been given a shortacting benzodiazepine such as temazepam. This is very efficient and has little or no hangover effect so that the players feel fine the next morning. The players take a late breakfast between 10 a.m. and 11.30 a.m. and are allowed to take whatever they want or feel comfortable with. Most tend not to eat a great deal, preferring cereal, but it does differ widely. Some, usually prop forwards, have a voracious appetite, irrespective of the time of day or night.

Around 12.30 p.m. a team talk begins, with the coach going over a few last-minute details dealing with the game plan. Then it is time to assemble on the team coach to take us to the national stadium. Over the years it is our experience that the journey to the stadium produces the first significant increase in adrenaline flow. This continues until well after the match is over.

The team arrive at the dressing-rooms and make their own preparations for the game, aided by the physiotherapist and the team doctor in attendance. It is at this point that one becomes aware occasionally of the psychological pressures that may prey on individual players. Team motivation (particularly in a physical contact sport such as rugby) may be undertaken to its greatest effect at this particular moment. (I have taken my own pulse on several occasions whilst in the players dressing-room and ten minutes before the kick-off it has always been over 120 beats per minute — and I was not even playing!) The players, needless to say, are at a peak of arousal for psychological motivation. Some captains and coaches are tremendous motivators with their team talks. Whatever the approach, the players are very susceptible at this moment in time and those with motivational problems or perhaps excessive competitiveness can, on rare occasions, channel this into excessive aggression. This has led to ugly scenes in the first few minutes of a game on some occasions over the years.

The newcomer to the international scene, very often, is susceptible to an anxiety state which can impair performance. This is where communication through a personal introduction to the players in a sympathetic and welcoming tone can prove very beneficial in helping to put the newcomer at ease. Many players chosen to play for their country are found wanting at their début. It is often debatable whether they are physiologically and psychologically capable of moving into the 'overdrive' gear that separates the very good club player from the international. Physiologically they may or may not possess the additional qualities required at international level. Psychologically, if they are too anxious, then their output of energy may be misdirected, causing them to perform below their best.

Violence, foul play and the laws of the game

In considering psychological pressure at international level, the overspill effect of motivation in the extreme situation of the international stage has been discussed. Unfortunately, these social symptoms are manifest in a more florid form in certain types of personality. In physical contact team games they may move from team to team, usually because of their antisocial behaviour both on and off the field of play. Mercifully the game itself usually tends to weed these players out, and it is made known to them that they are unwelcome. The real danger lies in the psychopathic coach who will condone and even encourage such players, and will nurture unfair tactics and techniques involving intimidation of the opposition. This may result in aggressive and antisocial behaviour in the team as a whole. Thankfully this has not been the author's experience at international level. The persistent offender is normally penalised out of the game and punished accordingly. In 1978 a rugby injury survey published in the *British Medical Journal* (Davies & Gibson 1978) highlighted the incidence of Rugby injuries as a direct result of foul play. This was produced by personal interviewing of injured players partaking in the survey by the author. Almost 30% of the injuries were attributable to foul play, but the significant factor was that only a quarter of the injuries attributable to foul play were penalised by the referee. Some time following its publication, the four home unions introduced a new law whereby, at senior and international level, linesmen were allowed to adjudicate and bring to the attention of the referee any misdemeanour which the referee obviously had not seen.

This is perhaps a very good example of the way in which the medical profession may, through a scientifically performed survey, isolate risk factors in a sport and persuade the sports governing body to implement fundamental changes in the laws of the game to improve safety.

Since the 1970s several injury surveys in rugby union football have been undertaken, looking at injury trends in the game and in particular the incidence of serious cervical spine injuries. In January 1988 a paper in the *British Medical Journal* entitled 'The need to make Rugby safer' by Burry & Calcinoi from New Zealand showed that cervical cord damage is a known hazard of rugby, and that changes in the rules of the game have been accompanied by a dramatic fall in the number of such injuries in New Zealand. This paper met with much support but also a good deal of criticism.

There is no doubt, however, that the medical profession can contribute very considerably in assisting the organisers and administrators of the game of rugby football to make it safer and more pleasurable to play. Burry & Calcinoi state in their paper that a decision was made in April 1987 by an Australian court to award more than A $2 million damages to a youth who became tetraplegic after an injury sustained in a rugby league scrum collapse. The judge castigated the State Government for failing to make known to the player and his coach the fact that players with long necks were much more vulnerable to cervical injury and should not be allowed to play in the front row of the scrum. Since the administration were known to be aware of this view, they were found to be negligent in not disseminating warnings.

Burry & Calcinoi conclude their paper by stating that a recent comprehensive study of cervical spinal cord injuries in various football codes in Australia found that in rugby union most injuries occurred in the 'collision phase' of scrum formation (Taylor & Collican 1987). As this danger can be eliminated be requiring the opposing front rows to engage and stablise themselves before the remainder of the players take up their positions, legal action could be taken against the administrators of rugby union by any player who damages his cervical spine during the formation or collision phase of a scrum. Failing to alter the rules of a game, despite the knowledge that existing practices were hazardous and that a safe alternative existed, could well be held by a court to constitute culpable negligence. The gauntlet has been taken up by the United States Rugby Football Union who in May 1988 held an International Injuries Conference in Boston, organised by the United States Rugby Football Union Foundation, a charitable trust. Speakers from as far afield as Wales, New Zealand, Canada, Japan and developing nations discussed injury problems. The main theme, however, which emanated from the conference was the very serious dilemma in which the USRFU could find themselves if they were held liable in a similar situation to that which had happened in Australia. Rugby Union is not played in schools in the USA, but is only taken up at the age of 18 or 19, on leaving high school. Previous playing experience for the vast majority is in American gridiron football, and players are therefore at risk when they encounter different tackling techniques, and especially through late introduction to scrummaging. With over 250 000 players participating every weekend across America, the game is rising in popularity, but is in grave danger of being sued out of existence if every effort is not made to ensure that adequate safety factors are both acknowledged and implemented. The role of the doctor here is to promote information through research.

Random dope tests are held following each five-nations international rugby game and to date there have been no positive results.

Being an amateur sport, rugby union football players are perhaps far less likely to expose themselves to the risks of drug-taking than are their counterparts in the professional code of gridiron football, where in the USA cases of cocaine and marijuana abuse have been widespread.

Conclusions and recommendations

In concluding this chapter on the role of the team doctor in international rugby, the author hopes that most of the issues related, both in anecdotal terms and on the subject of scientific research, convey the fulfilment that can be obtained from this privileged post. It is obviously necessary to have a profound knowledge of the game to fully achieve the greatest satisfaction from what at times can be an exhausting but nevertheless enjoyable position.

The post demands the commitment of long hours throughout the season, attending squad training sessions in the worst of British winter. The returns, however, are great; the camaraderie of rugby folk results in many good and lasting friendships throughout the world with like-minded individuals who enjoy this, probably the best of all amateur team sports.

In considering recommendations, I have touched not only upon the drugs question, but also on the laws of the game, and how these have been altered and may be further amended to avoid or at least reduce serious injuries.

To avoid major litigation which could seriously harm the game internationally, the International Rugby Football Board should be kept appraised of developments, conferences and medical research that seek to identify the risks in order that hazards may be nullified. It is within the power of the governing body of the sport, by so doing, to make the game safer and more enjoyable for all.

References

Burry & Calcinoi (1988) The need to make Rugby safer. *British Medical Journal*
Davies & Gibson (1978) Rugby injuries survey. *British Medical Journal*
Taylor T. K. F. & Collican M. R. J. (1987) Spinal cord injuries in Australian footballers 1960–85. *Medical Journal of Australia* **147**, 112–8.

The role of the physiotherapist in club and international rugby football 4

K. MURPHY

'Go not for every grief to the physician ...'
G. Herbert from *Jacula Prudentum*, 1651

Introduction

Medical cover for sporting events has historically been somewhat disorganised with irregular availability of expertise and experienced health care personnel. Much credit is due for work done by trained first aiders and the St John Ambulance in providing front line assistance to injured players on the field of play, but it should be recognised that organised attention by fully trained health care professionals is now demanded quite legitimately at higher levels of play. Despite the amateur status of a game such as rugby football, the level of professionalism and commitment displayed by the players means that injuries may be potentially severe and that, furthermore, players expect and properly demand that their injuries will receive the best possible attention from the time they are incurred through to full rehabilitation and resumption of activities.

In rugby union football, the continued developments of the leagues and the ever increasing demand for player excellence means that clubs have found it is important to have access to a suitably qualified physiotherapist as part of their front line service and also as a back up to training and rehabilitation.

Professional requirements

Nowadays it is important that the physiotherapist is professionally qualified rather than an enthusiastic amateur who, to quote one, informed me that he 'did not practice during the week as he had a "proper" job to do then'. The physiotherapist should be thoroughly professional in their therapeutic, managerial and counselling skills and should have a strong personal affinity and enthusiasm for the game, and for those players who come under their charge.

The physiotherapist should be well versed in orthopaedics and trauma with a sound background knowledge of medical and neurological conditions. Familiarity with neurology gives the practitioner much confidence in the ongoing re-assessment of stubborn injuries. The use of models for strapping practice is to be recommended, whilst the experience of being strapped oneself can

25

be a worthwhile educational process. Knowledge and practice of emergency resuscitation is an essential skill and should include the ability to intubate a patient where indicated, although this should be learned only under medical supervision.

It is helpful if the physiotherapy practitioner has first-hand experience of the game to which his or her professional services are offered, although for many female practitioners the absence of this opportunity is not necessarily a handicap. It is important, however, that the team physiotherapist should empathise with the treatment requirements of a player. Such qualities are unfortunately not always appreciated in the minds of certain club administrators who, whilst perfectly dedicated to their purpose, are sometimes rather tunnel-visioned.

Some years ago, a player, having injured his shoulder, sought early treatment so as to be fit for his club's cup match the following Sunday. Examination revealed a bruised deltoid rather than any serious joint injury and I felt confident in reassuring him that with treatment he should be able to play. When he returned on Monday his condition was improving and he was cheerful. Tuesday, however, found him forlorn and it transpired that the chairman of the selectors had said that injured players had to pass a fitness test on the Wednesday evening or face automatic bar from selection. The club in question was playing in the semifinal of their County Plate competition. The player, an experienced lock-forward, was desperately disappointed to see his chance of glory being denied and to make matters worse the chairman of the selectors was a back! We discussed it and concluded that the test could only be done in the evening inside the club house as they had no floodlights at that club. We opted for two further treatment sessions in the next day and discussed strapping of the injury but felt that this could prove to be counterproductive. Finally, with the deadline approaching and the injury still causing some problems such that he would be unlikely to pass the test (although I was confident he would be better by Saturday), I suggested that we strap the good shoulder and that he should do the test with this revealed under a vest. On Thursday a beaming and happy player appeared, the psychological effect of outwitting a back producing an even more rapid reduction in the remains of his inflammation. He played on the Sunday in the final and the chairman of the selectors at that time now attends for treatment!*

Participation in competitive team sports facilitates understanding of the motives which cause players to strive for selection: the hardness of training, the highs and lows of winning and losing, the

*This anecdote demonstrates admirably the quality of relationship that should exist between the health professional and the 'patient' where the interests of the player are placed ahead of the inflexible bureaucracy of officialdom. Medical paternalism is obviated by ensuring that the patient is fully appraised of the potential risks of premature resumption of play (see Chapter 1).

satisfaction of good decision making, the disappointment of injury and the tedium of recovery. Complete understanding of these ingredients will help the physiotherapist in dealing with the different aspects of recovery.

Roles

It is generally agreed that the main role of the team physiotherapist is to treat injuries but the importance of their role in the prevention of injuries is becoming increasingly appreciated. Working alongside doctors, manager, coaches, fitness advisors, selectors and administrators, the physiotherapist helps to ensure that the risk to players in training and in matches is minimised. This takes time, discussion and appreciation of the role of all parties within the infrastructure of the game.

Prevention

The fact that certain athletes spend up to 80 minutes preparing to run for under 2 minutes should be contrasted with the fact that some rugby teams spend 2 minutes preparing to run for 80 minutes. First-class teams now aim to be at the match venue at least an hour before kick-off and have time to prepare themselves by 'warming up'. Invariably, players who suffer muscle pulls blame their lack of warming up before playing. The purpose of the warm up is to produce an increase in overall circulation in conjunction with an increase in body temperature. All major joints in the body should be fully mobilised and those muscles acting across those joints should be stretched to their full extent, producing full extensibility and readiness for optimum contraction. This process is extremely worthwhile and should not be rushed. It is possible to lose players with pulled muscles from the warm-up if rigorous activity is attempted too rapidly from cold. Physiotherapists are involved in this work daily and their expertise should be sought in devising and leading such stretching routines prior to any physical session.

In the 1983 Lions tour after discussion Jim Telfer afforded every encouragement to myself as team physiotherapist to take the squad for 30 minute periods prior to every training session and it is worthy to note that no player suffered a pulled muscle until the last match of the 12th week of a physically demanding tour.

On the 1989 Lions tour Ian McGeechan and Roger Uttley allowed me as team physiotherapist complete freedom and encouragement over warm-up preparations. Again there were no withdrawals during the tour from muscle pulls and this compares favourably with Lions tours prior to 1983 when no team physiotherapist was taken.

Warm ups can be followed by remedial sessions for those recovering from injury so that the affected individuals may work using non-injured parts. They are thus still part of the squad and may take part in the talk-ins and are immediately available for treatment when the full squad complete their session.

Dressing-room rituals

The hour or so before the game should follow an organised and well-rehearsed pattern from the physiotherapist's point of view. It is assumed that the team physiotherapist has full knowledge of past and recent injuries of the players and also knows their requirements for strapping or padding with respect to these injuries. Acquaintance with a new team member and their requirements should have taken place well in advance of the dressing-room situation. Frequently members of the team like to take a stroll to acquaint themselves with the idosyncrasies of the pitch prior to the match. At this point I organise my work area. The value of a portable collapsible folding couch is well worth the problems of transport that it presents when travelling. To have a firm working surface for your height is as sensible for the physiotherapist as players having the correct size boots. A clean towel over the couch adds that clinical professional touch.

Convenient to the couch and set out in an orderly fashion a selection of the following should be available:

Elastoplast	7.5 cm (×4), 5 cm (×12), 2.5 cm (×8)
Rigid tape rolls	2" (×3), 1½" (×3), ½" (×2)
Pre-wrap rolls	(×2)
Vaseline tubs	(×1 large)
Embrocation tubes	(×3)
Vick	(×1)
Scissors	(×3)
Orthopaedic felt	5 mm × 1 sheet
Smelling salts bottle	(×1)
Variety of dressings	Primapore various sizes, ribbon gauze
Insulating tape	(×2)

I have found it unwise to put everything on show as somehow all items will be used. A few Elastoplast rolls and a pair of scissors are essential requirements to be carried in the physiotherapist's own pocket. All strappings should be applied before becoming involved in massaging (often termed 'rubs'). Rubs can range from stimulating to sedative and can often incorporate a passive stretch to the end of a range of movement with some active work for a muscle group that is giving some anxiety.

Although it may be more 'clinical' to use an adjacent medical room or area personally I prefer to work in the actual dressing-room area.* Firstly, the players are all together in their preparations and cautionary advice to an overenthusiastic 'do-it-yourself' strapper could avoid circulatory difficulty later in the game. Also there is the obvious time saving in change-overs between players and thus a greater opportunity to pick up and treat minor clinical problems such as skin abrasions that otherwise could well be ignored by the player. The captain and coach are still able to have their individual words with the players and not miss out any of them.

Field of play

While final preparations are taking place I make sure that I am properly attired with adequate layers of clothing suitable to the weather conditions. They must allow me to move freely enough to perform any necessary duties. I then check the medical kit bag that I will carry on to the pitch in the event of injury.

The medical kit bag will include:

1 Airway
Elastoplast   5 cm (×3), 2.5 cm (×3)
Rigid tape rolls   2" (×1), $1\frac{1}{2}$" (×1), $\frac{1}{2}$" (×1)
1 tin PR spray
1 small Vaseline
1 tube embrocation
1 small hand mirror
1 solid rubber gag
2 dozen gauze swabs
4 packets of Kaltostat
1 smelling salts
2 pairs of scissors
1 cervical collar
1 water bottle
1 waterproof container for sponge in iced water plus 2 small plastic bags of ice cubes
1 hand towel
Space or pocket for carrying spare contact lens sets, pair of laces
I also have charge of a spare shirt and shorts

The airway is necessary for any emergency resuscitation where a player is unconcious and the physiotherapist should be trained when and how to insert this. Fortunately it has to be used only rarely but it is a life-saving item.

---

* Strict principles of confidentiality may be dispensed with in the context of the pre-match dressing room. Time honoured traditions of team togetherness constitute 'volenti' unless a player indicates an express wish to observe confidentiality.

Elastoplast and rigid tape is used for emergency strapping of an injured joint or a contusion which is not severe enough to require the removal of the player from the field of play. At times this tape can be used for covering up or occluding an abrasion or cut which is not severe enough to warrant immediate stitching. Occasionally tape has found use for holding the sole of a boot to the upper where no spare is available although this is a rare scenario in first-class rugby.

PR spray acts as a surface coolant producing reflex analgesia following trauma. It should only be used, however, when there is no broken skin. I prefer to use an ice-and-water-cooled sponge, hand applied with some compression.

Vaseline is used to protect a cleaned graze or contusion where there is no blood leakage, especially round the eyes or ears.

Embrocation for a 'rub' may be requested by a player at half time to satisfy a muscle anxiety.

A small hand mirror can be of help to contact lens users in replacing a dislodged lens but its main use is to reassure a player about the size of a facial abrasion or bruised lip.

The solid rubber gag can be bitten by a player suffering from a seriously painful injury once over the initial shock and when awaiting a stretcher for removal from the pitch.

Gauze swabs are produced in the event of any blood leakage and are used for compression and cleaning purposes to reveal the injured area and so help in deciding whether a player should be removed from the field for attention or whether 'on field' attention may be adequate. The continued use of communal sponge and water on leaking cuts and abrasions should be discouraged for reason of cross infection, even though the risk of transmission may be low (see Chapter 8).

Kaltostat is a very effective aid to blood clotting and can be moulded into a nasal plug should this be needed.

The cervical collar may prove useful as a temporary supporting measure once serious cervical injury has been eliminated.

A hand towel has obvious uses but can also be used as a signalling device to attract the attention of the doctor or the replacements in the event that the player's injury is serious enough to cause him to withdraw from the field.

The spare shirt and shorts have obvious uses but there is now a further need for spare shirts to be available. In the event of haemorrhage onto the injured player's shirt or onto a fellow player's shirt both need to be changed, especially if the blood-stained area is likely to come into contact with an open wound on the player or opponent. At this time I find it useful to mentally rehearse the procedures I will go through when dealing with different injuries. This is also a double check on the contents of my medical bag.

Since 1988 changes in the Rugby Football Union (RFU) regulations allow an injured player to receive attention on the field of play whilst the game continues. This places added responsibility on the physiotherapist who now has to be tactically aware as well as medically aware. The physiotherapist needs to know the injured player's position and his importance to the team plan at the time of injury and has to ensure that the approach made to offer assistance to the injured player does not interrupt the flow of play. The injury must be rapidly assessed and an effort made to inform other players who may not yet have noticed who is out of action. It is important not to be in a vulnerable position when a change in the pattern of play occurs although this is sometimes very difficult to avoid. Finally, the physiotherapist should attract the referee's attention if the clinical situation so dictates.

The process of resolution of soft tissue injury should commence as soon as the physiotherapist commences his attention to the injured player. Inspection and enquiry before touching the injured part should be the order of the examination process. This procedure is of necessity restricted by force of circumstance but it should not be hurried although it should take somewhat less than 2 minutes. The instant and indiscriminate application of a dripping wet cold sponge should be discouraged particularly if there is bleeding. At inspection the physiotherapist should observe the amount of pain expressed by the player. Lack of movement or stillness is often an indication of a more serious injury than is dramatic writhing of a player on the floor.

Information about the injury and the player's sensation at the time of the injury should be obtained by direct enquiry of the patient. In considering prioritisation of actions to be undertaken a patent airway is the first consideration and the removal of the player's mouth guard is essential if there is any suspicion of head or neck injury.* Such injuries form a category of their own and require extreme care in their management and use and also demand use of specialised equipment and techniques. The assistance of experienced personnel should be awaited if any doubt exists and the game should be stopped immediately by attracting the attention of the referee.

Following inspection at the site of injury, having eliminated any serious misalignment or immediate swelling suggesting fracture of the injured part, the player should be asked if he can move the injured part himself. Assistance in the form of passive movement can be given which can lead on to assisted active movement. Assisted movement of the injured part and active movement against gravity should then lead to assisted weight bearing and subsequently to full free weight-bearing movement.

* Following any form of concussion the medical recommendations of the Rugby Football Union should be observed and the player must take a 3 week break, and furthermore must be fully neurologically examined by a qualified doctor before resumption of play.

The firm application of an ice-and-water-cooled sponge on the painful area at this time should counteract pain and facilitate movement. Satisfactory performance and return to full function should allow resumption of play while inadequate or partial recovery should cause the player to withdraw from the field for more detailed examination.

Treatment of the acute stage of soft tissue injury

It is well established that the pain, swelling and associated muscle spasm resulting from a soft tissue injury show an excellent response to ICE: 'I' for the physiological benefits of ice, 'C' for compression and 'E' for elevation and exercise.

Ice is best applied crushed and held within a damp towelling envelope, though any cold source, from cold tap water through to a packet of frozen peas is beneficial.

Compression may be applied to the injury by means of a bandage or Tubigrip, though I favour the use of a cylindrical garment which can be zipped, closed over the ice envelope and attached to an intermittent compression machine where it is subjected to rhythmic inflations (compression) and deflations (relaxation) or mechanical massage for a period of up to 20 minutes.

Elevation should take place during the application of ice and compression, when regular, rhythmic isometric contractions to the muscle groups superior to the injured part should also be performed.

The application of a firm supportive pressure bandage or full Watson–Jones type pressure bandage to the area plus non-weight bearing and elevation with exercise following ICE as a repeatable routine over the first 24 hours will have a beneficial effect on accelerating the resolution of the inflammatory process.

This will then lead into the remedial re-education stage of treatment where limited activity of the injured part can be encouraged and the unaffected limbs exercised to maintain overall general fitness, aiding psychological as well as physiological recovery.

Fitness to play

As recovery takes place and activity is increased the player asks the all-important question, 'When can I train? When can I play?' If possible, each stage of rehabilitation needs to be supervised. It is very difficult to predict recovery but certain signs and symptoms can help especially if the physiotherapist in the assessment actually saw how the injury took place. Was it sudden and dramatic? Was it gradual and protracted? Was there loss of function? What was the length of time before function returned, and what was the rate of improvement over the first 48 hours? These are the important questions to be answered.

Ultimately it is the player who declares himself fit but he can be assisted by repeated assessment and measurement of strength, flexibility and function in the affected part during recovery. If the pain and swelling can be removed and the player can recover the strength to control the increasing mobility of the injured part and can achieve full co-ordination he can normally return to squad training to improve fitness. Many factors play a part in the selection of an injured player who declares himself fit, notably the personality of the player, the relationship between the management, player and medical team — the importance of the game for which selection is intended and its timing in relation to other important matches in the season.

From club to country

Although players seen and treated at club level will sometimes appear at higher levels for county or country and may have the same type of injuries requiring treatment the circumstances at higher levels of play are significantly different with regard to provision of physiotherapy services. Furthermore, at all senior levels of play there has been a marked increase in awareness of the medical requirements and paramedical back up that clubs will now be expected to make available to their players.

The physiotherapist liaises with the team doctor about the medical condition of players, and the adequacy of medical provisions, and with the selectors about the availability of injured players for fitness testing, for training and for match selection.*

If a player requires a prolonged course of treatment he or she may well attend the physiotherapist's place of work. Continuity of treatment is very important to the on-going relationship between the physiotherapist and the injured player. The physiotherapist is in the best position to see an injury happen, be involved in the initial assessment and treatment and assist in the rehabilitation and return of the player to training. The interruption in continuity can sometimes retard recovery, although in the absence of an organised structure to provide medical care for players discontinuity of care is often what happens.

Paradoxically this may be the case for players at the highest level of play. An injury to an international player occurring in a Saturday club match will involve the immediate attention of the club physiotherapist. The national team physiotherapist may give attention that evening and the following Sunday morning. The player may subsequently seek attention from his own 'private' physiotherapist before falling back into the hands of services

* Issues of confidentiality between the physiotherapist and 'patient' in principle are the same as for the doctor–patient relationship. A qualified disclosure of information may be possible, however (see Chapter 1).

* The Access to
Medical Records Act
which came into force
on 1st November
1990 will provide that
disclosure of medical
records will be made
on demand after that
date.

provided by the club or national scheme. He may therefore encounter three or more different philosophies at various stages of recovery. This can lead to conflict within the treatment programmes devised by the various professionals involved which may prejudice the outcome of treatment. The initial hours after injury are probably the most critical with respect to the outcome of treatment and it would be helpful if the notes describing the treatment given were to be made available to the player if he was likely to obtain further treatment from another source(s) in the foreseeable future.*

Speedy recovery of an injured player is further enhanced by a close professional relationship with the club doctor, good medical facilities available at the ground and the co-operative attitude of administrators.

It should be remembered that although the final whistle signals the end of the game it usually signifies the start of the club physiotherapist's working week. During the close season the club physiotherapist may help in the monitoring of fitness of players, helping to pinpoint weakness caused by injury and providing a programme of specific exercises and precautions to be taken to prevent injury.

Physiotherapy at national team level

The following is an account of my experiences as the honorary physiotherapist to the England and British Lions rugby teams.

I feel that my commitment begins once the squad is announced. I may phone a player who has been omitted or a new cap if I know him. I will scour the papers and teletext looking for any reports of injured players and may phone them before they phone me. Liaison is formed with a number of club physiotherapists who keep me informed as to the progress of international players they may have treated.

The squad will meet on the Saturday evening the week before a match and thus an opportunity arises for players to approach me about their injuries and their need for treatment. The player will be examined and assessed by the team doctor and myself and treatment commenced as appropriate. A clinical decision following this examination may mean that training is contraindicated for an injured player and thus treatment will take place whilst the remaining members of the squad train. Team manager and coach have to be informed of the situation and prognosis in order to be able to decide on replacements. Injured players are encouraged to attend as it is always possible to give two or three treatment sessions at that critical stage.

Prior to the Sunday morning session, which usually starts on the pitch at 10 a.m., treatments, strappings and rubs are fitted in between breakfast and team meetings. Further assessments and strappings take place and once the coaching session starts I return to treat the players who are too injured to join in that session. Team work between the team doctor and myself is of paramount importance. Over the next 2 days injured players may contact me for advice, especially those who may not be in a position to get to their own physiotherapist. We meet again on Wednesday for a 9.30 a.m. start when the position of any injuries needs to be reviewed with the doctor, manager and coach. Any doubts about a player's fitness that the management might have are usually resolved by a thorough clinical assessment, review of the player's performance during warm up and also a review of his performance during a fitness test devised by myself.

If it is felt that a further 24–48 hours of treatment will bring about a return of full function then the full commitment in training will not be expected and the player may not take part in the sessions. Thursday usually has the squad assembled by 09.30 a.m., changed and ready to leave for training at the end of the team meeting. The strapping of most players will have been completed by then, and all I have to do is prepare for the warm-up, and with the doctor, be available during the training for any emergencies that arise. Should an injury take place and need more than on-pitch attention, then myself and the player will be driven back to the team hotel to start treatment. During the rest of the day I will be available for any additional treatments required by players.

Friday follows a similar pattern to Thursday.

On the Saturday morning of the game I am available to provide the final treatment sessions that players may need. The forwards and backs have mid-morning meetings and some like to come afterwards for a mobilising 'rub' before getting ready to depart for the match. During meeting time I make sure all my records of injuries and treatments are up to date, then I have the chance to check out my kit and pack my bags ready for leaving. Usually, all the medical kit has to be packed and taken to the match venue as well.

The hour before the match in the dressing room follows a similar pattern to that described earlier, the difference being that the atmosphere is vastly more charged at the highest level. When the match is over and the injured need attention I am always acutely aware that action taken at this stage can help the speedy resolution of an injury. Reassessment and treatments may need to be carried out on the Sunday before the players leave for home. These regular few days together bring the doctor and physiotherapist into close company and there is great opportunity to bring each other up to date on new procedures, techniques, drugs and equipment that may help the players. We can quiz each other about certain players' injuries, the mechanism, treatment and recovery and generally educate each other about improving and setting high standards of care and prevention within the rugby scene. The post of physiotherapist to an international union is held in an honorary capacity.

Touring

In my view, touring is the ideal situation in which to practise physiotherapy. England and the British Lions produce a squad of the fittest and best rugby players in the United Kingdom and the responsibility of the physiotherapist is to try to make sure that every one of them is available for training and selection. They are under the care of the physiotherapist 24 hours a day and if injured they want to recover as quickly as possible. One of the major advantages of touring as a physiotherapist is the fact that there is full continuity of care from the acute stage of injury through to rehabilitation. The majority of tours are now of 1 month's duration and involve seven matches. The Lions tours have been reduced from 3 months to 2 months and from 18 to 12 matches. There is therefore very little time tolerance for injuries and emphasis is on recovery, for if a player misses a week this represents three matches missed. Nowadays there is no realistic possibility that an injured player can be allowed to stay on the pitch 'just to see how it goes'. It is far better for the player to miss part of a match but to be available for selection for the next match especially early in a tour. If a player suffers concussion he has to come off and in view of the 3 week rule his tour is effectively over and a replacement has to be flown in. In the modern game there is a great pressure to gain results, especially at the highest level, which in turn places demands on medical staff to ensure that players are in their best condition possible to play. A week on tour is like the ground extension of a domestic international week but involving 30 players. With a continual change of venue (twice a week) the consequent travelling can be quite fatiguing. It always seems to be the case that, following a test match, the departure time the next morning is usually around 8 a.m.

Managers and coaches are under pressure to produce results and may get overtaken by media hype. Regular meetings between management and players should help balance the hard physical training necessary with game strategy. On tour, treatment of injuries has to be arranged around meals, training sessions, squad meetings, visits, trips, receptions and even matches. The treatment of injuries by physiotherapy must take precedence over all other activities in order that players may be presented in the best possible condition for selection. Records of injuries and treatments should be kept automatically, and with proper precautions to maintain anonymity comparisons between previous and recent tours can be made. This naturally provides the basis for research into mechanisms of injury and optimum methods of treatment to provide the quickest possible recovery. For example, by introducing a simple change in technique in the case of treatment of inversion injuries of the ankle I was able to show a reduction in recovery time from 13 days to 7 days during the 1983 Lions tour.

Summary

The roles, duties and responsibilities of a team physiotherapist within rugby union are far reaching and, in common with many situations, depend on the personality of the incumbent. In view of the fact that the proportion of female to male chartered physiotherapists in the United Kingdom is 9:1 it should come as no surprise that a number of first class clubs now have a female physiotherapist to provide this service. This is a welcome development. These individuals are a growing band of highly qualified people and although working in a male-dominated environment administer treatment in a most discreet and professional manner. I know that these services are greatly appreciated by the players.

Over the years it has been my experience that it is the players themselves who have upgraded the role and importance of the team physiotherapist. The players have first-hand knowledge of their commitment and skills. The physiotherapist forms a special relationship with the injured player in their lowest and most painful moments and may gain considerable professional satisfaction from seeing that player return to full activity in the shortest time possible.

5 Sports medicine and the law

EDWARD GRAYSON

'The Law fills gaps which the world of sport can never reach'

Prologue

The law linked collectively to medicine and sport was the last thought in my mind as a law student, after the Second World War had just ended, when the gross mistreatment of a simple fibula fracture from a mistimed tackle in the Oxford University soccer trials ended my active participation forever in the game, as a player. It led indirectly to a love for the law blending with a lifelong enthusiasm for all sports and thinking, writing and ultimately practising law as applied to sport.

Initial thoughts in that direction were developed with topics which the medical world in a sporting context may never need to contemplate. They were fired by dining in the Hall of Exeter College (where Britain's first organised Athletic Meeting and Club were formed in 1850 and nearly a century later Sir Roger Bannister dreamed of breaking the four-minute mile barrier), beneath a portrait of Mr Justice Eve. He had pioneered the concept of sporting educational charities with a High Court judgment delivered during the First World War. It confirmed a former schoolmaster's bequests to Aldenham School for the purpose of building Eton fives courts or squash rackets courts and an annual athletics school sports prize. In *re Mariette* [1915] 2 Ch. 284 was a landmark decision which the House of Lords unanimously endorsed 65 years later in the Football Association's Youth Trust Deed decision of *Inland Revenue Commissioners* v. *McMullen* [1981] AC 1.

That inspiration for sporting–legal thoughts led to published explanations after commencing practice at the Bar in the *FA Bulletin* and *Rating and Income Tax* during 1953 on the taxation anomalies between professional cricketers' tax-free benefits from public subscriptions and those of professional footballers which were then contractually based and thereby liable to income tax. They were followed by an abortive attempt to argue the now well-established restraint of trade principle in a county court case on behalf of Ralph Banks who had played against the immortal Stanley Matthews in

Ch: Chancery (Law Reports)

AC: Appeal Cases

This chapter is an updated version of that appearing in *Medicine, Sport and the Law* (1990) ed. S. D. W. Payne, Blackwell Scientific Publications, Oxford.

38

the celebrated Coronation Year FA Cup Final of 1953 when Black-pool beat Bolton Wanderers 4–3 (*Aldershot Football Club* v. *Banks* (1955) *Aldershot News* **4**, 25 November 1955).

Medical issues never surfaced at all during that period, although the personal suffering from that self-inflicted soccer injury was a classic case of *volenti non fit injuria* (he who voluntarily consents to lawful injury risks cannot claim compensation damages for it). It is correctly qualified by my co-editor Professor Bernard Knight's contribution on p. 165. Deliberate criminal and civilly actionable breaches of playing law nullify it. My broken fibula, when my foot stabbed the hard Iffley Road ground, tackling for a ball already whisked away by my opponent, illustrates it perfectly. Subsequent negligent hospital treatment, which created a legal liability, was sufficiently remedied elsewhere by specialist skills to deflect parental thoughts from the available compensation claim against the local hospital authorities.

Yet four decades later, when Butterworths' *Sport and the Law* (with 15 chapters and 10 appendices) took shape in the later 1980s, the chapter headed 'Sports medicine and the law' was the first to be written because its subject matter was then uppermost in my own and the general public's minds. It has contributed to the structure of the pages which follow. For the intervening years have developed this area of the application of the law to medicine within sport into the most important for sport in particular and society in general. It affects all sections of the community from the cradle to the grave as the national concept of sport for all becomes synonymous with health for all.

As a member of the editorial board I have had the opportunity and privilege to obtain an overview of all contributions to these pages, and thus to identify a pattern which emerges that is common to all the differing sporting disciplines where legal involvement cannot be ignored. They can be conveniently summarised as follows:

1 Any medical or paramedical practitioner in this growth area, as evidenced by our contributors, clearly has, or should have, an enthusiasm for his or her particular sports discipline.

2 Different sporting categories demand different levels of medical experiences and awareness and action, often in an international context. Yet as Dr F. Newton says at the end of his chapter, 'Medical hazards of water sports — and how to avoid them', in respect of the profile of the team doctor, with words of general application, it 'is much that of the old-fashioned family doctor.'

3 The medical adviser must always keep in mind the overriding duty to the individual performer as an individual patient.

4 Conflicts of duty between responsibility to the athlete patient and any governing or managing body should be recognised, identified and resolved in favour of the overriding professional duty

to the patient, and liaison should be established, if required, with the patient's more permanent GP. This position is comparable to the in-house industrial and commercial practitioner's relationship with employees (while being alert to the potential differences created between ambitious athletic achievers and/or their administrators desiring and, indeed, perhaps demanding, for competitive or individual participation, a medical opinion for fitness which conflicts with the patient's individual welfare).

5   There is a necessity for medical advisers to administrative governing, managerial, organisational or promotional bodies to:

(a) understand, identify and, if necessary, record their own legal relationships and areas of legal ·control and responsibility as contractors or agents;

(b) where appropriate, advise on suitable facilities and equipment, including communication with associated or back-up services for supplying appropriate medical action for every occasion; and

(c) recognise and act upon an entitlement to withdraw from any commitment if such advice is not pursued effectively, thereby placing such advice at risk for potential legal liability.

6   A requirement for keeping or logging adequate records for future reference in case of disputes over diagnosis and treatment may appear to be self-evident, but in circumstances of sporting medical emergencies this benefit to both patient and doctor may be overlooked.

7   There is a general across-the-board absence of adequate statistical information for assessing the extent of sporting injuries and levels of seriousness in order to gauge the problems which require the most immediate remedial action.

8   A precise definition of relationships and responsibilities and cross-communication is essential, if time permits in writing, between all parties concerned in respect of the sports doctor's appointment to act for an individual, team or governing body, for the purpose of accepting or avoiding a duty of confidentiality to an individual athlete or participant.

These common denominators emerge as the most apparent features which bind all the different sporting medical requirements in a common interest. Furthermore, the number of additional examples and citations which have been specifically identified in my own text here as having been incorporated while these pages were being prepared for the printers during the autumn and early winter of 1989, after its earlier structure based on the Butterworths' *Sport and the Law* publication in January 1988, demonstrates beyond doubt the rapid development of a growth area. It is illustrated almost daily, and indeed, inevitably, as the sporting world expands its horizons internationally to every corner of the world. Against this background, what follows here is an attempt to explain, within the limitations of space as comprehensively as possible, how the law and medicine can combine to benefit not only sport and its personnel in general, but also society, which all three disciplines should seek to serve. The laws are stated as at May Day 1991.

41

Chapter 5
Sports medicine
and the law

Table 5.1 A summary of Court cases resulting from sports injuries.

Date	Injury	Issue	Court	Case
1878	Ruptured spleen fatality from soccer tackle	Criminal manslaughter prosecution: Acquittal	Leicester Assizes	*R. v. Bradshaw* [1878] 14 Cox CC 83
1898	Internal injuries causing death from violent soccer jumping at opponent	Criminal murder prosecution: Conviction manslaughter	Leicester Assizes	*R. v. Moore* [1898] 14 TLR 229
1901	Fatality from boxing blow	Test case prosecution: Acquittal	Central Criminal Court	*R. v. Roberts* [1901] *Daily Telegraph*, 29 June
1968	Fatal blow causing death during niggling dispute in local league Essex soccer match	Criminal manslaughter prosecution. Convicted. Sentence: conditional discharge	Maidstone Assizes (transferred from Essex Assizes)	*R. v. Southby* (1969) *Police Review*, 7 February, p. 10
1969–70	Broken leg from foul tackle in local league Sussex soccer match	Civil assault (trespass to the person) damages claim: £4000 damages award and costs	Lewes Assizes and High Court, London for damages award	*Lewis* v. *Brookshaw* (1970) 120 NLJ 413
1977	Broken leg from foul tackle in local league Cornwall soccer match	Civil assault (trespass to the person) damages claim: £4000 damages award and costs	Bodmin Crown Court	*Grundy* v. *Gilbert* (1977) *Sunday Telegraph*, 31 July
1978	Fractured jaw in two places from off-the-ball punch in club rugby union match in South Wales	Inflicting grievous bodily harm contrary to s. 20 Offences against the Person Act, 1861. Convicted. Nine months' suspended sentence	Newport Crown Court	*R. v. Billinghurst* [1978] CLR 553

(1978 *British Medical Journal*, December, contributions: J. P. R. Williams and B. McKibbin, J. E. Davies and T. Gibson)

Date	Injury	Issue	Court	Case
1980	Fractured jaw, nose, cheekbone during 'friendly' rugby game	Inflicting grievous bodily harm contrary to s. 20 Offences against the Person Act, 1861. Plea: Guilty. Six months' custodial imprisonment (reduced without reasons on appeal to two months' custody)	Croydon Crown Court and Court of Appeal	*R. v. Gingell* [1980] CLR 661
1983	Head butt causing broken nose and black eyes to 38 years old local player in local league match	Civil assault (trespass to the person) damages claim: £400 general damages and £5.80 special damages and costs	Kingston County Court	*Hewish* v. *Smailes* (provided from court archives by H. H. Judge John A. Baker, DL)

Table 5.1 (Continued)

Date	Injury	Issue	Court	Case
1984–5	Broken leg from foul tackle in local league Leamington Spa soccer match	Negligence claim based on 'reckless disregard of plaintiff's safety which fell far below the standards which might reasonably be expected in anyone pursuing the game'. £4000 damages awarded and confirmed on appeal	Warwick County Court and Court of Appeal	*Condon* v. *Basi* [1985] 2 All ER 453
1985–6	Concussion from punch in off-the-ball rugby union incident	Guilty plea to common assault. Sentence: One month's custodial imprisonment reduced without reasons to one month's suspended imprisonment	Newport Crown court and Court of Appeal	*R.* v. *Bishop* [1986] *The Times*, 12 October
1986	Ear bite after tackle in police rugby union match	Inflicting grievous bodily harm with intent contrary to s. 18 Offences against the Person Act, 1861. Convicted. Six months' custodial imprisonment. Confirmed on appeal	Cardiff Crown Court	*R.* v. *Johnson* [1986] 8 CAR (S) 343
1988	Broken jaw by professional soccer player in tunnel after match	Guilty plea. Inflicting grievous bodily harm contrary to s. 20 Offences against the Person Act 1861. £1200 fine £250 compensation and costs	Swindon Magistrates' Court	*R.* v. *Kamara* (1988) *The Times*, 15 April
1988	Broken checkbone caused by amateur rugby player in club match kicking opponent on ground during course of play	Conviction: grievous bodily harm 18 months' imprisonment	Bristol Crown Court	*R.* v. *Lloyd* (1988) *The Times*, 15 September
1988	Broken jaw by amateur soccer player in 'friendly' match	Actual bodily harm	Wood Green Crown Court	*R.* v. *Birkin* (1988) *Enfield Gazette*, 7 April
1988	Damaged ligaments to professional footballer	Negligence claim based on illegal tackle. Agreed damages £130 000	High Court London	*Thomas* v. *Maguire and Queen's Park Rangers* (1989) *Daily Mirror*, 17 February
1989	Broken thigh and back injuries in fall caused by horse crossing in front of two other runners under guidance of jockey	Civil assault and negligence claim resulting in damages of $A121 490	Australian Supreme Court (Mr Justice Finlay)	*Frazer* v. *Jonst* (1989) *Racing Post*, 19 May, 26 May
1989	Concussion from kick on head to player on ground by soccer opponent	Grievous bodily harm. Eighteen months' custodial sentence. Confirmed on appeal	St Albans Crown Court and Court of Appeal	*R.* v. *Chapman* (Court of Appeal Crimimal Division transcripts)
1989	Kick during course of play to opponent causing two nights in hospital adjudicated to have been deliberate on spur of moment	Civil assault (trespass to the person) damages claim: £400 general damages; but claim for aggravated damages refused	Basingstoke County Court	*Vermont* v. *Green* (provided by Mr Oliver Wise, Barrister)

Table 5.1 (Continued)

Date	Injury	Issue	Court	Case
1990	Broken jaw from foul professional rugby league tackle	Civil claim assault for damages. $A 68 000 awarded against player and club	New South Wales Common Law High Court	*Rogers* v. *Bugden and Canterbury Bankstown Rugby League Club* [1991] *Open Rugby*, May, p. 56
1991	Broken neck from swimming dive	Civil negligence against Interalia Amateur Swimming Association	Nottingham Crown Court	*Nottingham Evening Post* [1991] 7 February

All ER: All England Reports. CAR: Criminal Appeal Reports. CLR: Criminal Law Review. NLJ: New Law Journal.

Introduction and issues

The role of sport within the international community was described by Professor Sir Ludwig Guttman in 'Reflections on sport in general' in his *Textbook of Sport for the Disabled*, published in 1976, with words which are as true now as they were when he wrote, 'Today sport plays an ever-increasing part in the life of the individual, as it does in the life of nations, and represents as much a positive element in the culture of our modern life as it did in the culture of ancient nations.'

The survival of sport on the public stage through sponsorship caused one of Britain's best known and experienced commentators, the late Ron Pickering, to address British sport's governing bodies at the Central Council of Physical Recreation's (CCPR's) annual conference at Bournemouth in 1985 with the following citation from the *Observer's* leading sports writer, Peter Corrigan: 'Sport took its soul to the pawnbrokers so long ago that finding the redemption ticket is not going to be easy.'

Four years later, in early 1989, that redemption ticket emerged at an international medical congress on injuries in rugby and other contact sports, organised by the South Africa Sports Medicine Association, within a heartbeat of where Dr Christiaan Barnard pioneered the internationally acclaimed first successful heart transplant operation at Cape Town's Groot Schur Memorial Hospital. For if medicine and music spell out an international language known to all peoples of the world, which transcends or should transcend all known barriers, so, too, does sport, and the injuries and damage to health that it can cause. Indeed, by 1990 the Central Council of Physical Recreation which represents all the sporting governing bodies in England thought fit to publish its *Fair Play in Sport: a Charter*, which is represented by permission in Appendix 5.1 at Page 83. It has been translated into 12 different languages.

In two crucial areas, violence and drugs (sport's own VD problem), medical services and their associated disciplines such as physiotherapy, pharmacology and biochemistry can alone identify the causes for which the law, in and out of sport, should be able to provide the remedy. Correspondingly, if medicine and its ancillary services err, the law provides areas for redress, particularly in the field of negligence and even, in the most extreme circumstances, through criminal liability.

Within the drugs scenario, doctors, pharmacologists and biochemists and laboratory staff have uncorked the bottles from which have poured the disagreeable evidence of cheating and attempted cheating by artificial stimulants. No less disagreeable, and of equal actual and potential consequence, is the other form of sporting injury to health: violent foul play. Curiously, and for reasons connected with long-established sporting mores and customs, linked to the macho image of robust play, any notion of cheating by physical injury has hitherto been underplayed, if not ignored: with increasing frequency throughout the world an offender or an offending team gains an unfair advantage over and against the victim through breaches of playing laws. This can also create breaches of national civil and criminal laws which merit intervention by traditional legal processes, in addition to sporting institutions and governing bodies'. disciplinary tribunals.

Thus sports medicine involves not only traditional treatment and availability of facilities, it is also a guide and reflection on the state of play according to sporting rules and laws or breaches of them. This was evidenced as long ago as 1978 when two crucial sporting medical contributions to the *British Medical Journal* (December 1978) identified medical evidence which crystallised respectively the injurious consequences of existing playing laws which required amendment and the civil and criminally liable consequences of undoubtedly violent foul play in breach of existing playing laws. J. P. R. Williams, surgical registrar, and Professor B. McKibbin, in the Department of Traumatic and Orthopaedic Surgery at Cardiff Royal Infirmary, warned in an article entitled 'Cervical spine injuries in Rugby Union football': 'Referees and coaches should be aware of the dangers of scrum collapses, especially as it seems to be an increasingly popular tactic to bring about this purposefully.' J. E. Davies, Research Registrar, and T. Gibson, Consultant Physician, recorded in an article entitled 'Injuries in Rugby Union football': 'in a prospective study of 185 players attached to 10 British rugby clubs . . . foul play might have caused as many as 47 (31%) of all reported injuries. Complete eradication of deliberately dangerous play would considerably reduce the high incidence of injuries in this sport.'

These two complementary examples of a common denominator for health hazards illuminate ideally the relationship between sports medicine and the law. They would also appear to reflect to this particular non-medical editor and contributor one of the factors which influenced the first Lord Horder in his early days at Bart's at the turn of the century, as explained in the memoir by his son entitled *The Little Genius* (1966): 'that preoccupation with the post-mortem room ... and an examination of the body after death was often, as it sometimes still is, the only way to arrive at the truth about a particular case, to confirm or upset a diagnosis, and to push forward the frontiers of knowledge in general. There is no arguing with the corpse on the slab.' A corollary to this appears in the current and 13th edition (1973) of *Glaister's Medical Jurisprudence and Toxicology*. Written initially by successive holders of the Regius Chair of Forensic Medicine in the University of Glasgow, John Glaister, Sr., and his son John Glaister, Jr., kinsmen of the BBC producer, Gerard Glaister, of such authentic television programmes as *Colditz* and *Howard's Way*, the Conclusions to the chapter entitled 'The medico-legal aspects of wounds' advise at p. 256 '. . . the examiner should direct his attention to the reconstruction of the cause of the injuries. He should first decide the instrument, then the degree of violence, the possibility of accident, the direction of the wound, and the relative position of the parties'. For sporting injuries caused by violent foul play this formula cannot be improved, and leads logically to the next citation from six years later.

In June 1979, after the British Medical Journal for 1978 cited above, P. N. Sperryn, in a paper to the British Association of Sports Medicine symposium, published in the *British Journal of Sports Medicine* (vol. 14, nos 2 & 3, August 1980, pp. 84–9), reaffirmed: 'It has recently become evident that deliberate foul play in certain sports is directly responsible for many sports injuries. It could be argued that the medical profession, on becoming aware of such trends in the style of play in sport, should be among the first to initiate the political changes which should lead to elimination of dangerous unfair play.'

No magic or new dimension exists for either medicine or the law in their application to sport. The law applies recognised criteria and principles to an area where it was traditionally recognised as a needless intruder until the complexities of modern administration and the intensity of modern competition demanded its arrival on a scene which conventional sporting sources were unable to regulate and control. The necessity for compulsory purchase orders and planning consents were as essential for the preservation and development of sporting premises as the necessity for courts of law to compensate victims and punish offenders of violent foul play.

More recently the nexus was highlighted in the sustained and extensive publicity in relation to the Sheffield Wednesday Football Club's Hillsborough Stadium disaster. In autumn 1989, in between Lord Justice Taylor's interim report (CM 765), published in August 1989, and his final report, published early in 1990, the recommendations, under the separate headings of 'Co-ordination of emergency services' and 'First aid, medical facilities and ambulances', are sufficiently comprehensive and relevant, in principle, not only to the tragic events which gave rise to this particular judicial inquiry, but also to all sports activities generally. Accordingly they are reproduced in Appendix 5.2. For the boundaries of sports medicine and the law are clearly not limited to playing areas.

So long as sport, leisure and recreational activities are capable of self-regulation, or careful or responsible control by sporting governing bodies or institutions or promotional organisations, without injurious or potentially injurious consequences, traditional legal sources are rarely required to intervene. When health and safety are at risk, the general legal system alone cannot protect the community which obtains its pleasures within the conventional sporting spheres. It not only needs evidence from the medical world, whether with regard to drugs, violence or maladministration, to prove specific breaches of regulations and of the rule of law with consequential health hazards. It also needs an awareness of the ethical and moral climate in which it operates.

Medicine as well as sport is caught up in the whirlwind of changing attitudes and scientific developments which demand decisions on many contentious ethical issues outside the sporting arena. Yet, as long ago as 1979, Sir Roger Bannister, from his standpoint as the first four-minute mile record-holder and neurologist before becoming Master of Pembroke College, Oxford, wrote in his foreword to Professor Peter McIntosh's book *Fair Play: Ethics in Sport and Education*: 'It is an increasingly popular notion among many young people that we can throw off ethical and moral principles in more and more spheres of life ... The fact of the matter is that we are faced with moral choices many times a day and if we do not notice them it must be that our intelligence or sensitivity is becoming blunted. Sport, which occupies the professional time of a few and the spare time of many, is a fit study for ethics.'

That study is beyond the scope of this chapter and of this book. Yet, as Bernard Crick, from his standpoint as Professor of Politics at Birkbeck College in the University of London, wrote in his preface to *Law and Morality*, edited by Louis Blom-Cooper and Gavin Drewry, in 1976: 'The structure of ethical arguments is hardly something to be determined *a priori* ... Both the fascination and the general problem today of the relation of law to morality — Does the law rest upon morality? Should the law concern itself with private morals? — arise because we no longer live in a society in which there is a clear moral code (whatever its basis) or in which there is consensus in the Ciceronian sense of common agreement as to right and interest.'

Nature nevertheless creates its own norm from the cradle to the grave. Medical remedies for healing and preservation of life have progressed down the years with new frontiers identified in succeeding centuries and generations: from Simpson with chloroform, Madame Curie with radiology, Pasteur with immunology, down to our own times with Banting, Best and Macleod with insulin and Chain, Florey and Fleming with penicillin. Yet, for the world of sport and its own capacity to operate as a mirror of and for society generally, medicine is the sole continuing area which can create a standard of awareness and recognition within the widest possible public for assessing tolerable or unacceptable conduct and attitudes. Within the context of this particular chapter, definitions and terms of reference to identify the areas affected are essential. Accordingly, attention will be focused on:

1 Definitions and terms of reference: sport, medicine and the law.
2 Violence and drugs (sport's own VD problem).
3 Medical intervention for women in sport and the law.
4 Medical standards and medical negligence.
5 Sport's future needs for medicine and the law.

1. Definitions and terms of reference: sport, medicine and the law

Sport

In Butterworths' *Sport and the Law* (1988) I cited two authoritative sources who independently arrived at the same conclusion from different points of the sporting compass. One was Sir Denis Follows, a wise and courageous administrator with three renowned sporting bodies: the British Olympic Association, the Central Council of Physical Recreation and the Football Association. In 1980 as Chairman of the British Olympic Association he effectively opposed Mrs Thatcher's embargo on the participation by British athletes in the Moscow Olympics staged shortly after Russia's invasion of Afghanistan. The other was the Director-General for many years of the Government-funded Sports Council, John Wheatley.

Before Follows died of cancer in 1983 he explained in a memorable Philip Noël-Baker Memorial Lecture at Loughborough College, 'I have reached the conclusion, after many years of trying, that sport defies definition. The Sports Council tried it and gave it up as a bad job.'

Two years later in 1985 during the course of a written Sports Council Memorandum to the House of Commons Environment Committee, which reported to the House of Commons in February 1986, based on the Council's conclusions under the title of 'Financing of sport in the United Kingdom', Wheatley stated: 'A study of the financing of sport produces a problem of definition. There is no single list of activities which would meet with universal agreement. Many years ago sport was felt by some to encompass hunting, shooting and fishing. A much wider view is now taken by many people.'

Indeed, with the television coverage of such diverse activities as darts, snooker and motor-racing, the time may well have come for a reassessment and re-evaluation of what constitutes sport, and particularly what sport is in relation to health and medicine. The *Concise Oxford Dictionary* traces its meaning derivatively to be an abbreviated form of the Middle English (1200–1500) 'disport' with various meanings, including 'frolic, gamble, enjoy oneself'. The celebrated Joseph Strutt in his book *Sports and Pastimes of the People of England, including Rural and Domestic Recreation from the Earliest Period to the Present Time* (1801) began his text with the classic claim, 'In order to form a just estimation of any particular people, it is absolutely necessary to investigate the Sports and Pastimes most generally prevalent among them.'

Nearer our own time during an address to the CCPR's annual conference in Bournemouth during November 1986, John Wheatley explained that, in the UK, participation in sport and recreation involved about 22 million in all 'on at least one occasion a month'. He added that 'Many of these, however, clearly do not see the need to join the governing bodies of sport, though their interests are affected by these governing bodies [which he numbered at approximately 390], which exercise some measure of control or guidance in the four countries of the UK.'

A great jurist, Lord Bryce, in his *Studies in History and Jurisprudence* (vol. 11, p. 181), observed that 'there are some conceptions which it is safer to describe than to attempt to define'. Sport is one of them. Hence Professor Sir Ludwig Guttman, in his *Textbook of Sport for the Disabled*, included among others this attempt by Unesco: 'Any physical activity which has the character of play and involves a struggle with oneself or with others, or a confrontation with natural elements, is sport. If this activity involves competition it must be performed with a spirit of sportsmanship. There can be no true sport without fair play. All rules must be observed with this in mind.' Within this context it is at least arguable that sport's function must include elements of health and education and risks within a self- or externally disciplined control; and those elements of control are essential to the manner in which the law and rules of play must apply to sport.

Legal

In the opening chapter to Butterworths' *Sport and the Law*, I have explained how *Britain: 1987*, an official handbook prepared by the Central Office of Information, explains at the beginning of Section

24, entitled 'Sport and recreation': 'The British invented and codified the rules of many of the sports and games which are now played all over the world', and within the sporting context they can be identified and categorised at four separate levels.

1 Playing laws: for players and participants to play. These are, in general, facilitative.

2 Penal playing laws: for referees and umpire to control and discipline play. These are, in general, restrictive.

3 Administrative laws: for fair and sensible organisation and control.

4 National laws: the overriding control for justice and fair play at all the above three levels.

They are extended by the international dimension in modern sport to two more widely embracing areas:

5 International governing body.

6 Overseas national laws.

I also illustrated their interaction by explaining that when a Welsh international rugby player in the autumn of 1985 punched a defenceless opponent during the course of a club rugby match without being seen by the referee:

1 There was a clear breach of rugby playing laws.

2 The player concerned was not disciplined by the referee in control.

3 The incident was ignored by club administrators.

Therefore as a last resort the national criminal law was invoked to the extent that a prosecution was launched for a criminal assault, which resulted in a conviction following a guilty plea. During the preliminary committal court proceedings, the chairman of Abercarn, Gwent, South Wales, magistrates' court on 13 May 1986 explained, 'It is difficult to decide where the rough and tumble of sport ends, and where criminality begins to appear in the game of rugby football. We therefore think the case would be more properly dealt with by a Crown Court.'

At the Crown Court, on a plea of guilty to common assault, David Bishop was sentenced to a custodial period of one month. A Court of Appeal reduced this to a suspended sentence for the same period. A month later, when this precedent was pleaded by counsel for an appellant who was a police officer who had been convicted of the offence of inflicting grievous bodily harm with intent (contrary to Section 18 of the Offences Against the Person Act 1861), and sentenced to six months' imprisonment for having bitten an opponent's ear when the two players were in close proximity immediately after a rugby tackle, Lord Lane, the Lord Chief Justice, commented that Bishop 'may consider himself lucky to have been treated so leniently.'

A few months earlier, in April 1985, a Court of Appeal in the Civil Division of the High Court affirmed an earlier County Court judge's award of £4000 damages to the victim of a foul soccer tackle in an amateur soccer match, resulting in a broken leg. The claim was couched in both negligence and trespass to the person, a civil assault, but the award was based on 'an obvious breach of the defendant's duty of care towards the plaintiff' (*Condon* v. *Basi* [1985] 2 AER 453).

In both illustrations the law of each game had been broken. The damage to the victim invoked the national law, too: in Bishop's case the criminal code, in Basi's case the civil code. On each occasion the complainant was a victim of a crime of violence, confirmed by medical evidence. Thus does medicine partner the law in illustrating Sir Ludwig Guttman's citation from Unesco, 'There can be no true sport without fair play.'

Sports medicine

An international publication, originating from Sweden in 1983 and first published in the UK in 1986 with the title of *Sports Injuries — Their Prevention and Treatment*, defined sports medicine as encompassing 'the following elements: preparation and training, prevention of injuries and illness, diagnosis and treatment of injuries and illness rehabilitation and return to active participation in sport. This definition relates to the athlete, the sport, sporting equipment and diagnostic instrumentation.' Each element in this area creates a potential legal issue and the definition must be regarded as incomplete unless the elements of administrative arrangements and provisions for their control and organisation, i.e. the responsibilities of promoters and employers, are included within or added to the final categories of 'sporting equipment and diagnostic instrumentation.'

One example has already been mentioned above: the recommendations for adequate medical services in the Sheffield Wednesday Hillsborough report, for which potential permutations of legal liabilities will be considered below (pp. 39–40). Another is illustrated by a vicarious liability which arose when Canadian courts awarded substantial damages against an employing club and doctors for rejecting complaints of serious sporting injurious consequences by a professional ice-hockey player suffered during the course of a game, explained in detail below on p. 37 (*Robitaille* v. *Vancouver Ice Hockey Club Ltd* [1981], 3 DLR 288).

DLR: Dominion Law
Report (Canada)

The strictly medical elements must be governed by the traditional and conventional legal sanctions within medical practice and its ancillary associations. Non-playing aspects such as sports equipment and diagnostic instrumentation are regulated by the general legal framework, which many people inside sport itself appear to be unaware can apply to the sporting scene equally as it does to the general community. Violent breaches of sporting laws and rules of play, condoned or inadequately disciplined by over-tolerant administrations, coaches, managers and referees, have created a misconception that sport could be a legal 'no-go' area on the basis that the law of the land stops at the touch-line or the boundary. How this is not the case is emphasised by medical evidence and clarified by the definitive manner in which the rule of law operates within a sporting context.

2. Violence and drugs

Each of these areas creates a cheating-at-sport situation. Violence is more clear-cut and identifiable. The issues of drugs in sport and how to deal with them can create confusion and injustice because of the overlap and, often, lack of communication between doctor, patient, administrator and lawyer. For violence there is no possibility of confusion. The only legal issue that arises is under what legal label violent misconduct in sport can be identified. Because of its comparative simplicity when contrasted with the complex administrative and medical drug scene, it may conveniently be dealt with first.

Violent sporting misconduct: the anatomy of foul play

This creates not only criminal and civil liabilities, but also claims for compensation from the Government-funded Criminal Injuries Compensation Board. It can also create ancillary contractual consequences, which, although not directly associated with medical issues, are nevertheless illustrative of violent misconduct. Thus in 1933 the Civil Court of Appeal in London reversed a trial judge's decision to reject a claim by an 18-year-old Irish heavyweight boxer, Jack Doyle, against the proprietors of the now demolished White City Stadium. He had forfeited his £3000 purse under the small print of the fight contract after the referee had disqualified Doyle for foul fighting in a contest for the heavyweight championship of Great Britain against Jack Petersen, now President of the British Boxing Board of Control. His lawyers had argued, because of their client's legal status as an infant, that the forfeiture was a legal penalty which was contractually disadvantageous and thereby not beneficial to their client. The test then, as now, under the Infant's Relief Act 1874, had been that an infant's contracts must be for beneficial necessaries. Lord Hanworth, one of Lord Denning's predecessors as Master of the Rolls, adjudicated, 'It is as much in the interest of the plaintiff himself as of any other contestant that there should be rules for clean fighting and that he should be protected against his adversary's misconduct in hitting below the belt or doing anything of the sort' (*Doyle* v. *White City Stadium Ltd* [1935] 1 KB 110).

All ER: All England
Reports
Cox CC: Cox's
Criminal Cases

The more directly actionable legal principles which have stood the test of time for over a century to outlaw violent sporting misconduct were reaffirmed as relatively recently as 1975 when the Court of Appeal Criminal Division in *R. v. Venna* [1975] 3 All ER 788 (p. 793 f–g) explained, '*R. v. Bradshaw* [1878] 14 Cox CC 83 can be read as supporting the view that unlawful physical force applied recklessly constitutes a criminal assault.'

In the Bradshaw case a jury acquitted a footballer who had been prosecuted for manslaughter after causing injuries during a friendly football match, no doubt because evidence was produced, from one of the two umpires in charge of the game, that no unfair play occurred. During prosecuting counsel's opening speech to the jury, Bramwell LJ interrupted a reference to the game's rules to say (p. 84), 'Whether within the rules or not, the prisoner would be guilty of manslaughter if while committing an unlawful act he caused the death of the deceased.'

The summing-up to the jury before its 'not guilty' verdict included these words, which with their references to intention and recklessness contain the key to both criminal and civil liability: 'If a man is playing according to the rules and practice of the game and not going beyond it, it may be reasonable to infer that he is not actuated by any malicious motive or intention, and that he is not acting in a manner which he knows will be likely to be productive of death or injury. But, independent of the rules, if the prisoner intended to cause serious hurt to the deceased, or if he knew that in charging as he did, he might produce serious injury and was indifferent and reckless as to whether he would produce serious injury or not, then the act would be unlawful. In either case he would be guilty of a criminal act and you must find him guilty, if you are of a contrary opinion you will acquit him.'

TLR: Times Law
Reports (as distinct
from *The Times*
reports)

Twenty years later, in *R. v. Moore* (1898) 14 TLR 229, the evidence had a stronger flavour with a stronger result. The accused offending footballer

1 jumped violently with his knees against an opponent's back;
2 threw the victim violently against a knee of the goalkeeper;
3 caused internal injuries resulting ultimately in death a few days afterwards.

The summing-up on this occasion to the jury by Hawkins J (pp. 229–30) explained: 'The rules of the game were quite immaterial ... it did not matter whether the prisoner broke the rules or not. Football was a lawful game, but it was a rough one and persons who played it must be careful to restrain themselves so as not to do bodily harm to any other person. No one had a right to use force which was likely to injure another, and if he did use such force and death resulted, the crime of manslaughter had been committed.... If a blow were struck recklessly which caused a man to fall, and if in falling he struck against something and was injured and died, the person who struck the blow was guilty of manslaughter, even though the blow itself would not have caused injury.'

After that verdict in 1898 no record of serious reported sporting violence from competitive as distinct from playground play has been traced for nearly 70 years until 1968. Then the crime explosion in society generally spilled over on to sporting fields, illustrated by the medical evidence provided ten years later by Davies and Gibson in the citation above (p. 45) from the *British Medical Journal* in December 1978 and subsequently by the Criminal Injuries Compensation Board. It was illuminated and high-lighted for all the world to see, as it can still see on telerecording films, as chronicled by one of the most renowned international athletes, the Brazilian soccer star, Pelé. In *My Life and the Beautiful Game* (1977) he has explained with Robert L. Fish, as I have narrated in Butterworths' *Sport and the Law* (pp. 205–206) citing Pelé and Fish at pp. 144–155, when identifying his experiences during the 1966 World Cup competition in Britain, '. . . against Bulgaria . . . I had been the target of merciless attacks from Zechev of Bulgaria throughout the entire game. Zechev did everything he could physically to cripple me, and the referee, Jim Finney[*] gave neither me nor any of the others on our team the protection we had a right to expect from an official in a game.'

'Morais, of Portugal, had a field day fouling me; eventually putting me out of the game. He tripped me, and when I was stumbling to the ground he leaped at me, feet first, and cut me down completely. It wasn't until I actually saw the films of the game that I realised what a terribly vicious double-foul it was. The stands came to their feet screaming at the foul, but the English referee, George McCabe allowed Morais to remain on the field, although again, even in the most inexperienced league in the world, he would have been thrown out for either of the two fouls, let alone both. Dr Gosling and Mario Americo came to help me from the field, and Brazil went on to play with ten men and ended up eliminated from the tournament.'

Those impressions of what the films showed for Pelé have been confirmed by my own viewing at least seven times of the nationally marketed official film of the 1966 World Cup Competition, *Goal*, by its scriptwriter and the *Sunday Times* football correspondent, Brian Glanville, and also by *The Times'* senior sportswriter, David Miller. The consequences legally are independently and interdependently the sixfold as set out at p. 49 above.

They were all repeated 14 years later during the semi-final of the 1982 World Cup competition in Spain. The West German goalkeeper Schumacher assaulted the French defender Battiston in a manner condemned internationally by the sporting press. Yet as David Miller recorded in his book on the 1966 World Cup, *The Boys of '66: England's Lost Glory* at p. 21, 'Any dignified sport would

[*] NB Jack Rollin, football's leading statistician and author of the *Guinness Book of Soccer Records*, in his *World Cup Triumph 1986* records the referee as Herr Tschenscher of West Germany . Pelé's text is as cited here.

have suspended for life the West German goalkeeper for his atrocious foul in the 1982 semi-final, which shamefully handicapped the French. From FIFA there was no more than a murmur.'

Battiston's 1982 experience against West Germany and Pelé's experience against Portugal and Bulgaria in the 1966 World Cup created a classic combination of circumstances which *could* and *should* have demonstrated — but did not — how all six legal layers acted upon and with each other in an effective policy because the fouls merited the following sanctions:

1 Sending off from field punishment.
2 In breach of Law 12 — violent conduct or serious foul play.
3 Suspension or dismissal from competition in the manner suffered 12 years after Pelé by Scotland's star winger sent home from the 1978 World Cup in Argentina following a positive drugs test in breach of FIFA rules but lawfully prescribed under Parliament's Misuse of Drugs Act 1971 (see p. 65).
4 National prosecution for assault occasioning actual bodily harm.
5 International governing body as in (2) above with censure upon referees and FIFA noted by David Miller for abdicating responsibilities.
6 Overseas national as in (3) above, with the precedents from other violent visitors or criminal offenders to visiting shores.

Nothing at all in fact ever happened. The offenders escaped back to their native lands without any effective punishment for their respective and undoubted criminality. The reluctance of the prosecuting authorities in the Liverpool area (covering Goodison Park where the Pelé assaults occurred) to take action could conceivably have resulted from diplomatic sensitivities. Since then, in the next World Cup, at Mexico City in 1970, England's captain, Bobby Moore, was intimidated by a false charge of alleged theft in the Colombian capital of Bogota; and as the world knows, 20 years later, the South Wales prosecuting authority charged the Welsh international amateur rugby footballer David Bishop with the offence identified and suffered by Pelé. It might well save rugby football from following the same slippery path to self-destruction taken by violent players and abject administrators at domestic and international levels. To those who supinely and irresponsibly say 'It's all part of the game', Pelé's beautiful game and that of others — the game of ballet without music — there is one question to be answered. What should happen to any member of a dance routine chorus whipping the feet from under the legs of Fred Astaire and Ginger Rogers? Punishment or condonement?

By 1980 the Criminal Injuries Compensation Board felt constrained to record in its paragraph 30: 'While there is now considerable public awareness of the existence and extent of football violence, we doubt whether the public is aware of the catastrophic effects which result from such criminal acts. The Board frequently deals with cases of people scarred for life, sometimes with cases of people seriously and permanently maimed and occasionally with people who are killed. We welcome the efforts which the courts, the police and many sporting organisations are making to attempt to lessen the number of such crimes.'

Seven years later, in 1987, the Board was still reporting (paragraph 37, p. 14): 'In the last few years, the Board has received an increasing number of applications arising from violence among players, particularly during rugby or football matches . . . We consider that it is in the interests of everyone that people who commit criminal offences on playing fields should be prosecuted. Anyone who considers that an injury upon him was caused by a criminal offence should draw the attention of the police to it. If he does not do so, he is unlikely to receive compensation from the Board.'

This last caveat identifies paragraph 6(a) of the Board's Compensation Scheme, which provides for withholding or reducing compensation for delay, non-disclosure to the police and other inhibitory factors. The criminal and civil pattern which has emerged is summarised in Table 5.1. The sample recorded represents only the tip of an ever-growing iceberg, the extent of which can never be fully known because of the absence of any means of collecting accurate data to gauge the range of the problem. This situation is well illustrated by a chance discussion while these pages were being prepared, with a former President of the Medico-Legal Society, Judge John A. Baker DL (a friend since our Oxford days) during a lull in court business at Kingston upon Thames. He enquired casually whether a judgment he had delivered in the Epsom County Court a few years ago for a soccer injury would be of interest and assistance. The response was positive, and the consequence now is that, to the list extracted below from Butterworths' *Sport and the Law* (and subsequent occurrences since its publication in January 1988), should be added the example which was unreported and embedded in the Epsom County Court archives until disclosed by this generous thought from the Circuit Judiciary with a very strong medico-legal association: disclosed in 1989, but relating to events in 1981, and heard at Epsom County Court in 1983.

While these pages were in preparation for the printers a chance meeting in the Temple with another practising barrister, Oliver Wise, produced yet another unreported case. This related to events at Basingstoke County Court in October 1989, in which he had been instructed before His Honour Judge Galpin, which precedes Judge John A. Baker's citation in the table below. Oliver Wise commented that his case which had been pleaded as a civil assault based on the tort of trespass to the person did not contribute to jurisprudence. Yet with Judge John A. Baker's precedent they each reflect a trend which was unheard of during our post Second World War Oxford days, but regrettably is being reproduced regularly in criminal courts at all levels as well as in the County Courts and High Courts to a degree which is unknown but cannot be ignored (Table 5.1).

In most of the examples in Table 5.1 the offences breached Rugby Law 26 or Soccer Law 12, which prohibits violent foul play, in addition to the civil and/or criminal law of the land. They are merely recorded examples of countless other less formally recorded examples throughout the world. Thus in 1985 a woman footballer who broke an opponent's jaw in a women's friendly (*sic*) soccer match on May Day was convicted of assault and ordered to pay £250 compensation by Clacton magistrates in Essex (*Baker* v. *Bridger* (1985) *Daily Express*, 1 May). And in 1986 from the USA an assault was reported which could have been prosecuted in the UK, arising from a fight between two women jockeys. One bit the arm of the other, who needed a tetanus injection. The stewards imposed a $30 fine for 'causing a disturbance in the jockeys' quarters', a TV room (Calder Race Course, Miami, *Daily Express*, 1 July 1986).

The wider British Commonwealth, however, from Canada and Australia has entered two areas yet to be pursued in the UK, vicarious liability for sports field injuries against *non-players*, as in the Canadian case of a claim against Vancouver Ice Hockey Club Ltd and its doctors (see p. 78). In another Canadian case, this time from British Columbia, and in a case from New South Wales, Australia, victims of broken neck injuries sustained in rugby scrums are suing respectively:

1 the opposing club, and, in the Australian case, the coach too;
2 the opposing/controlling Rugby Union;
3 the controlling referees' association;
4 the referee;

on the basis that they were vicariously responsible for the victim's injury through negligent control and administration. In the Canadian case the reference has exonerated and the Australian litigation was settled out of Court.

A more conclusive Australian case, however, decided at the end of 1990 and listed at the bottom of Table 5.1 has resulted in the first traceable judgment for vicarious field playing misconduct. It emerged from a foul tackle in an Australian rugby league professional match. The victim sued and obtained judgment against not only the offending player but also against the employer club. At the time of writing in early 1991 the club was reported to be contemplating an appeal.

A further traceable judgment for vicarious liability occurred in early 1991 when a former schoolboy swimmer obtained an apportioned damages award against a sporting governing body, the Amateur Swimming Association. He broke his neck when diving into a pool at the shallow end from starting blocks in 1983. At a trial in early 1991 at Nottingham Crown Court the Association was adjudged liable to an extent of 25% for his injuries (the remaining 75% liability being attributable to defective school training and instruction). It had not given sufficiently clear warning notices as one of the co-organisers of the event about the dangers inherent in the specific diving activities in accordance with the existing practice as at the date of the injuries in 1983, which has been amended since then but too late to avoid the risk at that time.

Also in the UK, the Scottish Football Association has disciplined two of its senior referees and downgraded the level of games which they can control because of alleged ineffective action against two fouling footballers, i.e. not dismissing them from the field of play: on one occasion when serious ligament injury resulted from an illegal tackle, and on another occasion for persistent dissent.

One frequent and insidious complaint about the national law entering into the realm of playing field illegalities is that sporting governing bodies can take care of it all. This, however, is not the case. For, separate and apart from inconsistencies in sentencing, they cannot, or at least do not, attempt to compensate a victim. Thus, when the Arsenal defender Paul Davis broke the jaw of the Southampton player Glenn Cockerill in full view of millions of television spectators during 1988 he was disciplined by an FA Commission which suspended him from playing in nine future games and imposed a £3000 fine. No one ever suggested by either inference or from facts that any money was paid to the victim. Yet two years earlier, when a Sussex County League player head-butted a referee, who was knocked unconscious, after the referee had penalised the offender, the victim consulted his local solicitor, Robert Rogers, who represents Sussex RFU on the RFU at Twickenham. The wise legal advice was to operate the Criminal Injuries Compensation Board's recommendations and place the matter in the hands of the police. A prosecution resulted. The charge of assault occasioning actual bodily harm was committed by local lay justices to Chichester Crown Court in West Sussex. The offender pleaded guilty. He was sentenced to 28 days' custodial imprisonment and ordered to pay £400 compensation to the victim. No sporting governing body would order compensation to the victim, recognising the legal vulnerability of doing so, and no governing body felt itself equipped to adjudicate and assess the level of compensation satisfactorily.

So far, to date, no known case can be traced for vicarious criminal prosecution against an administrator, coach, manager or other official. Logic and the spiralling developments as shown in Table 5.1, however, point inexorably in that direction if offenders do not desist from erroneously regarding bodily contact sports and other games as a licence to commit crime. This has been recognised in recent years by a pattern of awareness which can be identified from examples which may appear to have been isolated at the time but now form part of a consistent perspective. In 1987 the English Rugby Union Executive banned four players from selection after a Welsh international player, Jonathan Davies, suffered a broken cheekbone by a foul tackle creating an assault which was not prosecuted. FIFA has legislated for a mandatory red card for the assault which is inherent in the erroneously called professional foul, and the International Cricket Council has legislated for supervisory referees to oversee umpires following successive failures to outlaw intimidatory and potentially injurious fast bowling which also spills over into the area of assault. The Newcastle–Gosforth Rugby Union Club banned for life an international player with a consistent track record for field play misconduct. The Football Association penalised Arsenal and Manchester United financially and by deducting Football League points for public order offences, against which no appeal was lodged, and the Arsenal Directorate fined the team manager in an unprecedented disciplinary decision.

Such developments are consistent with an awareness that if the upward pattern of unlawful, as distinct from accidental, injurious conduct does not cease, then one day a criminal prosecution will be brought for aiding and abetting, counselling and producing such an offence against someone other than the offending player himself. If this sounds remote and beyond belief, it will be salutary for potential offenders to observe the words of Lord Goddard when Lord Chief Justice, a former Oxford University athletics half-blue and subsequently adjudicator in the inter-varsity Oxford–Cambridge athletics matches during his period of office in the 1950s at the now demolished White City Stadium in London. In 1951, with two other eminent judges, Humphreys J and Lord Devlin (as Devlin J) sitting in the King's Bench Divisional Court, they dismissed an appeal against conviction by a magazine proprietor of *Jazz Illustrated*, who had been convicted by Bow Street Magistrates' Court in London under Article 18(2) of the Aliens Order 1920 of aiding and abetting a breach of condition of entry into the UK of a greatly admired US citizen and musician, the jazz saxophonist, Coleman Hawkins. The basis for the conviction and its affirmation was that the offender had encouraged the breach by supporting a performance on stage. Lord Goddard emphasised that 'if he knew the offending proprietor had booed, it might have been some evidence that he was not aiding and abetting' (*Wilcox* v. *Jeffery* [1951] 1 All ER 464).

One of the generally unseen consequences of violent misconduct in the soccer scene was recorded in the *Guardian* on 18 November 1988 by its experienced football correspondent, David Lacey. He explained how 'Referees who officiate at football's lower levels are leaving the game in droves because of the rising number of assaults by players. The problem has become sufficiently serious for the FA to set up a special sub-committee to look into it ... There are 41 000 clubs in England, but only about 25 000 referees. Verbal abuse is bad enough but attacks on referees are running at more than 200 a session and the figure is rising.

After 230 assaults had been reported for the 1986–87 season the FA launched a referees recruitment drive but now, following prompting by the county FAs and the Referee's Association, they are going to give the matter a thorough investigation.'

Since those words were cited and while these pages were being prepared for the printers towards the end of 1989, rugby union referees have been reported requiring police protection publicly at renowned Rugby Union grounds after undoubted criminal assaults on referees; and thus the spiral of violence, especially against sources of authority, never diminishes. Many will recall the despair of the distinguished Metropolitan Police Chief Superintendant and referee, George Crawford, who felt obliged to walk off from refereeing what became fighting between two famous Rugby Union clubs during the mid-1980s. He now contents himself with adjudicating for school matches, where innocence can be protected if not corrupted by evil examples of public performers abusing great games as a vehicle and licence for criminal misconduct.

Before passing to the poisonous climate of the sporting drug scene, two final areas of sporting injuries require special attention. One has been confirmed by the London Court of Appeal since these pages were first formulated; schools sporting injuries, particularly for rugby, and insurance. The other is boxing and has been covered comprehensively in its medical and ethical context by the representative contributors from the amateur and professional disciplines (Chapters 18 and 19), and the Supervising Editor's note on the medical–moral arguments against the sport, particularly at professional level. The legal position of boxing has never been defined with certainty and finality for mainly historical reasons, and, as we shall see it is still developing. Parliamentary legislation in Australia, Canada and South Africa has attempted to regulate it. In Britain its only overall control is through the courts. The reported cases for over a century have moved from validating limited sparring as lawful (*R. v. Young* [1866] 10 Cox CC 370), via prize fighting until defeat from exhaustion or injury as illegal (*R. v. Orton et al.* [1878] 39 LT 293: *R. v. Coney* [1882] 8 QBD 534), to an acquittal of a manslaughter prosecution based on a fatality in the ring *not* caused by a boxing blow (*R. v. Roberts* (1901) *The Sporting Life*, 20 June, p. 8) and a bind over to keep the peace of the realm on the eve of a featherweight title fight (*R. v. Driscoll and Moran* (1911) *British Boxing Yearbook* 1985, p. 12).

In 1976, however, the Supreme Court of Victoria in Australia was required to formulate a criterion which ties in with the con-current opinions expressed by Drs Adams, Wren and Whiteson (Chapter 18), and a well publicised precedent which occurred while these pages were being completed for the printers in November 1989. Adams and Wren at page 243 explain: 'Regulations are only as effective as those who implement them ... Improving the standards of the referees and other officials across the country is a slow and difficult process, but over the years a steady progress has been maintained. A fact which may surprise those outside the sport, and is a source of concern for the medical officers within it, is that it is not a requirement for these officials to maintain a valid first aid certificate. The fact that many other sports are in a similar position does not make that any more acceptable.' Dr Whiteson corroborates this impeccable medical approach with his advice and important qualification (p. 281): 'Providing the medical education of all referees is adequate and constantly being updated, as it is in this country, then the referee, in the opinion of the author, should continue to be in sole charge of the contest.' That important qualification 'as it is in this country' was particularly significant in relation to the World Championship Title Fight at London's Royal Albert Hall during November 1989 between Azumah Nelson, the title holder, of Ghana, and Jim McDonnell, the challenger from Great Britain. The fight had been stopped in the twelfth round after McDonnell's right eye was badly injured and the events leading to this caused the respected and experienced columnist in the London *Observer*, Hugh McIlvanney, who is known for his sympathy to the boxing sport, to write in the issue for Sunday 12 November 1989; 'The fact that the challenger had fought with coolness, nerve, skill and energy through ten rounds (and seemed to me to be no more than a point or so behind ten at this stage) became heartbreakingly academic in the eleventh when his right eye closed suddenly into a ball of bruised flesh after what seemed to be a bang from the Ghanian's head. That injury represented a crippling handicap against a champion who, in spite of a largely torpid performance, had exhibited his famous capacity for havoc in the fifth round with a left hook that hurled a dazed McDonnell off his feet for the first count of his career ... Now began a series of misjudgments that could only provide encouragement for the abolitionist lobby. First, the referee, Joe Cortez, looked diligently into the sightless right eye and declined to intervene. Then, half-way through the eleventh, he did summon a Board of Control doctor, Ashwin Patel, to ringside to make an examination. From his home in New Jersey last week, Cortez said the doctor merely advised him to 'watch the eye' (ignoring it would have been some feat) and did not recommend that the fight should be stopped.

I find such a feeble response from the doctor incomprehensible; and the referee's contribution was underlined when he failed to endorse a stoppage after the first of two knockdowns in the twelfth.'

The potential significance medico-legally from Hugh McIlvanney's viewpoint was crystallised in the Supreme Court of Victoria. Mr Justice McInerney in *Pallante* v. *Stadiums Property Limited* (No. 1) [1976] VR 331 rejected a procedural application to strike out the statement of claim which formulated the documentary basis for a claim by a boxer who had received eyesight injuries when boxing under Australian Boxing Alliance Rules. He sued all persons other than his opponent, namely the promoter, his trainer, the matchmaker and the referee. The argument that the contest was a prize fight was the basis for the rejected application. The judgment as recorded in the summary of the report at p. 332 vindicated boxing as 'not an unlawful and criminal activity so long as, whether for reward or not, it was conducted by a contestant as a boxing sport or contest, not from the motive of personal animosity, or at all events not predominantly from that motive, but predominantly as an exercise of boxing skill and physical condition in accordance with rules and in conditions the object of which was to ensure that the infliction of boxing harm was kept within reasonable bounds, so as to preclude or reduce, so far as is practicable, the risk of either contestant incurring serious head injury, and to ensure that victory should be achieved in accordance with rules by the person demonstrating the greater skill as a boxer.'

The ultimate result of the claim was never disclosed, and in the absence of contrary information, should be treated as having been settled. Its existence as a live and modern precedent justifies and affirms the warnings and guidance built in to the contributions from Dr Adams, Wren and Whiteson in their respective contributions hereafter (Chapters 18 and 19).

A more clear-cut result occurred when the London High Court and Court of Appeal were required to consider an important schoolboy rugby injury case of significant consequence to all schools and their medical advisers as well as the victim.

The chronological sequence of dates (Table 5.2) is important for recognising and identifying the legal issues and consequences resulting from a policy decision by the Medical Officers' Schools Association (MOSA), and injuries suffered during an inter-house school match. This resulted in extensive litigation which, at the trial and on appeal, exonerated the school from coaching and insurance liabilities, but the medico-legal position is built in to the initiation and stimulus behind the underlying circumstances.

The action before Mr Justice Boreham lasted 26 days, and occupied 100 pages of a typescripted reserved judgment. Medical evidence relating to the injuries from a defective tackle blended with coaching evidence on rugby playing skills. Most significantly, the judgment relating to the insurance claim was based upon the principle that, because parents are under no obligation to insure, a corresponding duty cannot be placed upon schools. Since then, the Rugby Union has introduced a comprehensive scheme for rugby-playing schools under the terms of its Wavell Wakefield Charitable Trust, and the Central Council of Physical Recreation has pioneered a scheme on a wider basis.

The Van Oppen case raised many consequential legal issues not directly relevant to the medico-legal text, which I have discussed in the *New Law Journal* and also *Rugby World and Post* (*New Law Journal* **138**, 352, 29 July 1988 and *Rugby World and Post*, September 1988, p. 13 and [1989] 1 All ER 273: *Van Oppen* v. *Clerk to the Bedford Charity Trustees*). In this perspective, however, it is significant that MOSA identified issues which in turn had their own consequential effects of alerting the sporting world to the necessity for adequate insurance cover at every active level.

Table 5.2 Events surrounding the Van Oppen school-boy rugby injury case.

Date	Action
1979 July	MOSA recommended insurance for all rugby-playing schools
1980 November	Simon Van Oppen injured in the tackle
1981 July	Bedford School implements MOSA report
1988 July	Mr Justice Boreham in London's High Court rejects claim for damages compensation. The claim being based on two grounds: 1 alleged negligent coaching of rugby techniques 2 alleged non-insurance as recommended by MOSA report
1989 April	Court of Appeal dismisses appeal and confirms judgment

Accordingly, those behind the scenes who do not discourage violent sporting misconduct cannot say that this does not put them on notice; and, if the medical profession and its associated disciplines recognise the issues and alert their patients sufficiently, collectively, individually and at administrative and governing body levels, they can contribute as much to the elimination of cheating by sporting violence as they have tried to contribute to at least the control, if not the elimination, of drugs in sport. A report from the Council of Europe dated 20 July 1989 cited the International Olympic Committee as having stated through its own medical commission in Seoul that doping can be considered as one of the factors causing violence. The Council of Europe's report[*] stated, without identifying the range or area of sources, 'Six out of 10 football players asked in March 1989 thought that a direct relationship exists between doping and violence on the pitch', and then concluded: 'If doping generates violence, one way to combat violence is to eradicate doping, through joint actions, both preventive and repressive, between governments and sports bodies at national and international level.'

[*]Dr John O'Hara, the experienced Chairman of the Football Association's Medical Committee, has emphasised to me that ten years of random drug testing within the FA's jurisdiction have found *no* player guilty of *deliberately* taking drugs (see also pp. 27–28).

Drugs

No need exists here to explain the highest possible profile which the drugs scenario commands on the public sporting medical stage.

The Canadian Government inquiry into Ben Johnson's position and the much criticised attitudes of ambivalence of international athletics administrators at the Olympic Games and International Amateur Athletics Association, towards reinstatement of offenders against drug offences, are continuing issues at the time of writing. Another Canadian example and one from Scotland illustrate the problem which this particular area can create for doctors, administrators, participants and lawyers if the interaction between sporting regulations and lawfully prescribed drugs is not clearly recognised and defined.

An example of the necessity to understand clearly the true nature of the substances involved and their impact on sport and health was illuminated graphically during 1987 by a controversial public discussion about the use of beta-blockers. It was highlighted by a letter in the *Times* sports letters column from Dr I. M. James, Reader in Clinical Pharmacology at the Royal Free Hospital, Pond Street, NW3: 'A great deal of ill-informed comment has recently been voiced on the use of beta-blockers to obtain unfair advantage in certain competitive sports. The sports involved are those where the possession of a steady, non-tremulous hand is an advantage. No one has pointed out that, whilst all beta-blockers have an effect on heart-rate, only certain members of this family of drugs have an effect on tremor. Basically beta-blockers can be divided into cardio-selective, where the effect on a tremor is minimal, and non-selective, where the effect on tremor is marked. Certainly in the case of Neal Foulds a cardio-selective beta-blocker was chosen. This seems to me to be a very clear evidence of a desire in his case at least not to obtain unfair advantage.'

These two cases from Canada and Scotland demonstrate the need for harmonious communications between so many different but interlocking areas concerned with this very sensitive but crucially important medico-legal penalty area.

Ron Angus and the British Judo Association

In 1984 the *Sunday Telegraph* announced, according to information from the British Judo Association, that a dope test on Ron Angus, winner of the under 78-kilo category in the All England Championship in December 1983, had proved positive. A sample contained traces of the banned substance pseudoephedrine.

Angus, who had dual Canadian–British nationality, claimed that the substance must have been contained in a sinus decongestant which he had taken under a lawful medical prescription by his Canadian doctor. Yet, because he had breached the Association's requirements, he was banned for life from competing in British championships.

Five months later, after he had taken legal advice, the *Daily Telegraph* reported that the High Court in London had lifted the ban with the Association's consent. It admitted that the absence of a hearing for Angus to explain his position breaches the rules of natural justice, and the life ban was duly rescinded. The Association's rules have now been tightened to place the onus on competitors and by implication, therefore, on their personal doctors, to ensure that lawful medication does not contain banned substances (*Daily Telegraph*, 15 June 1984).

Willie Johnston and FIFA (Fédération Internationale de Football Association)

In a different set of circumstances, the communication issue in the case of Ron Angus is in principle not dissimilar from that of Willie Johnston, the former Scottish international soccer player who was sent home in alleged disgrace from the 1978 FIFA World Cup competition in Mexico. In his book *On the Wing* he explained how his own English Football League doctor lawfully prescribed Reactivan pills for his nasal condition. His national team manager has explained in *The Ally Macleod Story: an Autobiography* how the Scottish FA doctor clearly warned Johnston about drugs; but the footballer patient had not realised that the pills contained a stimulant.

After the result was known Macleod has explained that the Scottish FA doctor asked the player sternly, 'Did you take Reactivan tablets before the game against Peru?' 'Yes,' came the immediate reply. 'But you told me you didn't take drugs,' said the doctor, puzzled as well as angry. 'They aren't drugs,' was the astonishing answer, and Johnston went on freely to admit that he had taken them 90 minutes before the game, as he had previously done at club level with West Bromwich Albion.

'Incredible as it may seem, it appeared that Johnston, a man of 31, who had been looking after himself for a long time in the tough world of professional football, had missed the whole point of the doctor's repeated warnings. I have thought about the matter a great deal over the months, and it is my view that he really believed that his Reactivan tablets were little more than smarties,' writes Macleod.

Both the Angus and the Johnston cases demonstrate the need for clear comprehension and understanding by athletes of the nature of any lawfully prescribed stimulant, and of any potential impact upon a sporting governing body's own regulations. They also prove the necessity for medical advisers to try to establish that comprehension and understanding by the patient; and if justice is to be achieved by administrators they should heed the provisions of the British Parliamentary statutory defence under Section 23(3)(b)(i) of the Misuse of Drugs Act 1971, that any accused person shall be acquitted of a drug offence 'If he proves that he neither believed

nor suspected nor had reason to suspect that the substance or product in question was a controlled drug', i.e. one of which the use
is controlled by the Act, and thereby unlawful generally.

That sub-section, like others comparable to it in principle, is laid
down by Parliament, and illustrates the problems which face sports
participants who require drugs lawfully for medicinal purposes.

I have attempted to resolve these problems by posing the following questions in Butterworth's *Sport and the Law* and Sports
Council publications:

1   How are athletes and their personal doctors to know when a
breach or potential breach of a sporting governing body's rules
against drug abuse occurs?

2   How are sporting governing bodies to know that a failure to
meet their own stringent rules for the protection of a particular
sport does or does not arise from a lawful medicinal prescription?

3   How are lawyers to balance the interests of the sport in which
they advise administrators with the need to respect the rights of
individual competitors?

4   What is the patient to do when faced with what may become a
conflict of personal health interests against the undoubted right in
a free society to participate in healthy competition?

These questions cannot be shirked and have to be thought
through within the framework of what lawyers recognise, usually in
the international legal field, as a conflict of laws situation. Furthermore, with the explosion of international sport, and the concern of
the World Health Organisation as well as international governing
bodies about the problem, there is the added issue of international
harmony for approaching solutions.

Suffice, therefore, that we should begin at home in the UK, by
ensuring the following:

1   Doctors who treat patients competing athletically must familiarise themselves with the requirements of the particular sport
in question, both at domestic and international level and pass on
this information to their patients, the interested athletes.

2   Lawyers who advise administrators must see that any regulations to prevent cheating do not either transgress the rules of natural
justice and the opportunity to be heard, or contravene the spirit of
the British parliamentary defence that ignorance of the facts can be
a defence in a drugs case.

3   Administrators should try, together with doctors, pharmacists,
pharmacologists, lawyers and drug manufacturers, to attain a balance between the sport's rules and the individual's medicinal requirements, in the interests of fair play, health and the avoidance
of cheating.

4   Competitors must familiarise themselves with their own medical requirements within the rules laid down by their particular
sport.

As a last resort, because drug abuse is a national and international health hazard, the Government surely cannot opt out of taking an interest here, just as it is no longer ignoring its need to become involved with the problems of sporting crowd violence. As a start, consideration could be given to whether the lethal and recognised use of any known sporting drug substances, in addition to those which are already prohibited, should be outlawed alongside LSD, heroin, cocaine and other illegal substances. The proposal announced by the Home Office (in September 1987) that anabolic steroids were under consideration for being added to the lists of prohibited drugs is clearly a step in the right direction.

One long-term solution is offered by the Sports Nutrition Foundation which at present is housed in the London Institute of Sports Medicine under Dr Dan Tunstall Pedoe's jurisdiction at St Bartholomew's Hospital in London. It was created with the support initially of the Central Council of Physical Recreation, and its self-evident title points to a beneficial bodily health progression with long-term consequential effects. It does not and cannot claim to compete, however, with the short-term cheating advantages aimed for by drug takers.

Finally and by no means least in the never-ending struggle to reconcile bona fide drug medication with competitive sport, is the controversial impact of the contraceptive pill on the woman's athletic arena. Dr Ellen Grant in her challenging study, *The Bitter Pill: How Safe is the Perfect Contraceptive?*, published first in 1985, has explained how 'artificial derivatives of the male hormone testosterone are present in nearly all of today's pills' (p. 18, 1986 edition). The triple Olympic Games hurdler and Cambridge University blue, Peter Hildreth, commented in one of his *Sunday Telegraph* athletics correspondent's columns on 4 February 1986:

> 'There is evidence that women athletes who use it while not in breach of the rules are nonetheless reaping the benefits of illegal doping. The pill, a hormone, part of whose action is to reinforce the body's reserves at times of high physical demand, not only prevents loss of performance during menstruation, but also triggers a variety of advantageous side-effects. According to Dr John Guillebaud, author of the definitive textbook on the subject of the contraceptive pill, it stimulates an increase in the level of steroid hormone secretion from the adrenal and thyroid glands . . .
>
> 'In sport the pill has served its users not merely in its intended role of protection against conception, but also by suppressing menstruation, in tiding them over those difficult times when training or competition would otherwise be curtailed. There was a time when the unlucky coincidence of the cycle with championship dates was known to have a decisive bearing on medals. The arrival of the pill meant that one of the variables accounting for loss of form was effectively mitigated, if not banished.'

No doubt there will be arguments against such contentions for which no definitive answer and solution can be assessed. What cannot be doubted is that the creation of the pill and its side-effects on athleticism in women should at least be considered, if only to be reflected alongside all other elements which demand the closest and most balanced approach by everyone identified here. We should be concerned with the manner in which the correct harmony between sport, medicine and the law can enhance the health of the individual alongside performance in sport.

3. Medical intervention for women in sport and the law

Separate and apart from the possible impact of the contraceptive pill as a performance-enhancing drug, two current developments have given the medical profession a wider relevance to the position of women in sport since the days when Mrs Martha Grace at Downend, near Bristol, bowled her three sons, E. M., G. F. and W. G. Grace, to cricketing immortality in the mid-1850s, and the daughters of John Willes, the Kent professional of that period, are attributed with inventing round-arm bowling because their skirts impeded their underarm deliveries. One is medical — the sex change operation; the other is social — the equal opportunities legislation. Both categories have been covered in depth in Butterworths' *Sport and the Law* in the chapter entitled 'Women in sport and the law', from where much of what follows is drawn.

London's High Court in 1970 witnessed a then unique claim to annul a marriage because of the sex change operation, when medical evidence proved that the female party to the marriage had been born a man. In *Corbett* v. *Corbett (ors. Ashley)* [1970] 2 All ER 33 Mr (later Lord Justice) Ormrod, himself trained as a doctor before being called to the Bar, was asked to adjudicate on this then unprecedented condition. In acceding to it he held that the party who had undergone a sex change operation 'is not a woman for the purpose of marriage but is a biological male and has been since birth.'

Around that period, unknown to many outside family circles a distinguished writer, too, James Morris, underwent similar surgery to become Jan Morris; and five years later sport caught up with this new medical phenomenon in the year Parliament passed the Sex Discrimination Act. Dr Richard Rasskind, a New York ophthalmic surgeon, and a skilled tennis player, received similar surgical treatment to become after the operation Dr Renee Richards. Inevitably, the question emerged: what were the tennis authorities going to do about it? For the next two years Dr Renee Richards shunted between various US tennis tournaments which were sufficiently enlightened to accept her entries with the knowledge of her transsexuality. Those which were not, either rejected her outright, or conditionally upon chromosome tests being factually or conveniently satisfied. The world-wide International Tennis Federation invoked Olympic

Games tests which the doctor was unable to satisfy. When the locally based tennis authorities also required such stringent limitations upon entry the New York's jurisdiction was invoked. In an action against the United States Tennis Association, the US Open Tennis Championship Committee and the Women's Tennis Association Inc., during 1977, Dr Richards claimed relief as a professional tennis player who had undergone sex reassignment surgery which had allegedly changed her sex from male to female. She sued for a preliminary injunction against the organisations

1   to prevent reliance on a sex-chromatin test for determination of whether she was female and thus

2   to permit her participation in the Women's Division of the US Open tournament.

The legal foundation of the action was that the condition breached the anti-discriminatory code built in to the New York State equal opportunities legislation. After hearing a battery of conflicting medical and tennis evidence, Judge Alfred M. Ascione held: 'when an individual such as plaintiff (*sic*), a successful physician, a husband and father, finds it necessary for his own mental sanity to undergo a sex reassignment, the unfounded fears and misconceptions of defendants (*sic*) must surely give way to the overwhelming medical evidence that the person before him is now female'. Accordingly, a requirement that the plaintiff pass the sex-chromatin test in order to be eligible to participate in the tournament was grossly unfair, discriminatory and inequitable, and violated plaintiff's rights under the New York Human Rights Law, and granted the injunctions (*Richards* v. *US Tennis ASSN & ORS 1977*: 400 NYS (2nd) 267).

NYS: New York
Supplement (2nd
series)

Similar reliefs would have been available to Dr Richards at that time under British law if she had been subjected to similar conditions for a UK tournament. Not only could the Sex Discrimination Act 1975 have been invoked, as a result of the Court of Appeal's decision that acknowledged matrimonial sterilisation in *Bravery* v. *Bravery* [1954] 3 All ER 59 (where a wife failed to obtain a cruelty decree because the majority of the court held that she had consented to her husband's vasectomy), Dr Richards could have argued that the condition to undergo a sex-chromatin test would comprise an incitement to commit or to attempt to commit a battery.

By the time Dr Richards arrived in Britain, however, she came with an entirely different professional tennis status; as coach and adviser to the future Wimbledon champion, Martina Navratilova in 1977. This lasted for five years until Dr Richards retired from professional tennis and returned to her other profession, ophthalmic surgery. By then, 1982, English courts had begun to consider 'the average woman'.

In a different age group and in a different social setting a 12-year-old schoolgirl's wish to play soccer football with boys projected medical attitudes to women in sport via the Nottingham County Court to Lord Denning and Lord Justice Eveleigh and Sir David Cairns in London's Court of Appeal during 1978.

Section 44 of the Sex Discrimination Act as mentioned above contains the sole section identifying sport in a very limited manner. It comes within Part V of the Act under a general heading alongside other categories including charities, insurance and other circumstances nominated as 'General Exceptions from Parts II to IV', i.e. those covering employment, education and other unlawful discriminatory areas. It was enacted thus: 'Nothing in Parts II to IV shall, in relation to any sport, game or other activity of a competitive nature where the physical strength, stamina or physique of the average woman puts her at a disadvantage to the average man, render unlawful any act related to the participation of a person as a competitor in events involving that activity which are confined to competitors of one sex.' The key concepts here, of course, are the antithesis between 'the average woman' and 'the average man', and also 'competitors'. Both have been considered in the reported decisions of the tribunals and the courts. Both will doubtless have to be considered again. In a survey of the first decade's operation of the legislation from its inception on 31 December 1975, Lady Howe, the Equal Opportunity Commission's first deputy Chairman wrote in *The Financial Times*, 3 January 1986, 'The legislation was neither perfect nor comprehensive.' No reference was made to section 44. If it had been, the comment would have been justified that the first decade reflects an exploratory experience with a stop–go pattern. The reported cases illustrate a gradual move towards its beneficial application to sports women with the inevitable hiccups en route. Furthermore, a valuable survey by Dr Alice M. Leonard for the Equal Opportunities Commission of *The First Eight Years* (1976–83) (summarised in the *New Law Journal*, 31 January 1986) of the tribunal referrals identifies in its fuller text *sport* alongside 'Literary, artistic' in the applicants' occupations for claims under both the 1970 and the 1975 Acts; and for men as well as women only 1% of those who utilised the legislation are logged under these three comprehensive categories.

With such scant material no definable pattern can yet be traced; but the recorded cases in the various reported sources manifest a tentative approach bedevilled by the unrealistic delineation between 'the average woman' and 'the average man'. Women no less than men in sport demonstrate talents and qualities well above average which the slightest reflection can easily recognise. Indeed, this Parliamentary injection into sex legislation of the commercial shipping language of averaging suggests that the draftsman of the section and Parliament not only did not understand women in sport but could not have understood the above average skills which are the hallmark of true athleticism.

What is the 'average woman' and what is the 'average man' in *this* context has yet to be *fully* investigated by the courts. A tentative approach to it was made in the unreported decision of the Court of Appeal when it was concerned with whether or not a 12-year-old schoolgirl was discriminated against playing football with boys of her own age (see *Bennett* v. *The Football Association Ltd and The Nottinghamshire FA* [1978] CA 591). Tentative, because the issue and evidence called before the county court and accepted in the Court of Appeal was directed medically towards comparing and differentiating between boys and girls of 12 years of age, below and above the age of puberty; and a conclusion that the circumstances of the case proved existence of a disadvantage (the Act being silent on age levels). The playing merits do not appear to have been argued of the 12-year-old plaintiff-contender for a place in the boys' team for which she had been selected. Yet Lord Denning (at p. 2 of the transcript: no. 591 of 1978) said 'She ran rings around the boys'; and a witnes as recorded in *The Daily Telegraph* report of the county court hearing said she was 'a vicious tackler and once tackled a 15-year-old so hard he had to be supported and taken from the field'. This pointed, of course, to this particular plaintiff *not* being put 'at a disadvantage to the average' boy! Concentrating on what appeared to be a diversion in evidence from doctors about puberty, and without apparent arguments on above average skills, the Court of Appeal overruled the Deputy County Court Judge who had adjudicated and awarded £250 in favour of the 12-year-old 'vicious tackler' of 'a 15-year-old'. Two years later in *Greater London Council* v. *Farrar* ([1980] ICR 266), the Employment Appeal tribunal at p. 272 C–D per Slynn J said, 'we read the decision of the Court of Appeal as applying to the particular facts before it'.

ICR: Industrial Cases
Reports (sentencing)

Certainly the imbalance between the medical evidence concerned with puberty and the apparent absence of argument on the evidence tending to prove the existence of above average athletic talents which did not disadvantage the female plaintiff leave this decision without any general guidance for future disputes in the manner stated above; and any schoolgirl footballers not caught through average talents by the exclusion clause in section 44 can at least consider their chances on different evidence and arguments of a replay.

4. Medical standards and medical negligence

The ordinary principles applicable generally to medical liabilities operate within the sporting context, subject to two crucial general considerations. One is the absence of any traceable pattern of liability arising out of medical services in the UK which contain a sporting flavour. The other is a corollary to it: the general public's and even judicial misapprehensions about claims for sporting injuries which have been expressed during the last three decades.

The limited researches of practitioners would have been responsible for the following observations of Lord Diplock as Diplock LJ in a claim concerning a photographer injured by a competitor's horse in the White City Horse of the Year Show and by Lord Donaldson as Sir John Donaldson, Master of the Rolls, in the negligent tackling soccer case. In *Wooldridge* v. *Sumner* [1963] 2 QB 43 at 65, Diplock LJ noted: 'It is a remarkable thing that in a nation where during the present century so many have spent so much of their leisure in watching other people take part in sports and pastimes there is an almost complete dearth of judicial authority as to the duty of care owed by the actual participants to the spectators', albeit in the context of that particular case where a professional photographer was the injured plaintiff; and, in *Condon* v. *Basi* [1985] 2 All ER 452, Sir John Donaldson said (p. 453): 'It is sad that there is no authority as to what is the standard of care which governs the conduct of players in competitive sports generally and above all, in a competitive sport whose rules and general background contemplate that there will be physical contact between the players, but that appears to be the position.'

QB: Queen's Bench
(Law Reports)

Both statements are rebuttable by precedents which emerged during the years between the two World Wars from the realms of golf and motor racing: *Castle* v. *St Augustine's Links* [1922] 38 TLR 615 and *Cleghorn* v. *Oldham* [1927] 43 TLR 465 (golf); *Hall* v. *Brooklands Auto-Racing Club* [1933] 1 KB 205 (motor-racing); and *Brewer* v. *Delo* [1967] 1 Ll. Rep. 488 (golf). Nevertheless, this limited pattern emphasises the reluctance, in the UK at least, to invoke legal remedies for sporting injuries, during a period, of course, when the aggression inherent in modern competitive sport was less intense than it has become today, with the greater prize money and prestige that are associated in the manner identified in the chapter by Donald A. D. MacLeod.

KB: King's Bench (Law
Reports)
Ll. Rep.: Lloyd's List
Reports

Thus, the duty of care which a doctor and paramedical services owe to their charges, a breach of which alongside a reasonable foreseeable risk of injury or damage creates liability in negligence, should be recognised whenever a sporting injury requires treatment. The specialised medical sports injuries clinics and centres which are developing demonstrate a growing awareness of the need for such care. In these locations doctors are undoubtedly alerted to the obligation at all times to observe the risks within such a specialised sphere. Yet the risks may not necessarily be recognised or realised sufficiently or at all by the doctor or his associates, who may regard treatment of a sporting or sports-related injury by a casual or part-time participant, such as a sprained wrist suffered by a weekend golfer or tennis player, less seriously than that of an injured motorist or factory worker incapacitated from employment. 'You must give up golf, or tennis', is not unknown advice to such victims as the simplest treatment, without any recognition of the value of such activities to the patient and the long-term potentially dangerous consequences of such untreated situations. The weekend golfer or part-time cricketer with muscular ailments is no less entitled to the same level of medicine as any other patient; and the author's own legal and sporting professional experiences, information and observation confirm this trend among non-sporting medical practitioners who do not share their patients' sporting enthusiasms and interests.

Furthermore, the judicially recorded 'almost complete dearth of judicial authority' in the UK is not reflected in the more litigious climate across the Atlantic, as can be seen below; and this is compounded by the problems inherent in the evaluation of medical evidence, albeit for more complex general categories than those sporting medical science has produced in the courts so far. Recently, in *Wilshire* v. *Essex Health Authority* [1988] 1 All ER 871, the House of Lords directed a retrial with guidelines for the burden of proof because of judicial 'misunderstanding at the original hearing of evidence', and an 'irreconcilable conflict of medical opinion as to the cause of what was a complication in a premature birth, with substantial injurious consequences'.

A similar conflict of medical opinion associated with premature birth resulted in an earlier reversal by the House of Lords and the Court of Appeal of a £102 000 damages award, solely because the trial judge had drawn the wrong inferences of fact from the conflicting medical evidence. He had failed in the eyes of the appellate courts to distinguish between negligence and an error of judgement, for which no legal liability exists — the result in that case (*Whitehouse* v. *Jordan* [1981] 1 All ER 267). Together, these important House of Lords verdicts emphasise what Lord Scarman recorded in yet a third ruling from that ultimate judicial tribunal, as summarised in a contribution in the *All England Law Reports Annual Review*, 1987 (p. 179): 'What is remarkable about professional malpractice in the case of a doctor is that the courts have uniquely conceded to the medical profession the right to determine when there has been breach of that duty of care (*Sidaway* v. *Board of Governors of the Bethlem Royal Hospital and the Maudsley Hospital* [1985] 1 All ER 643 at 649).'

The areas within the sporting sphere where medical negligence can arise were considered in the chapter 'Sports medicine and the law' in Butterworths' *Sport and the Law*, taken from Butterworths' *Law and Medical Ethics* by Professor J. K. Mason and Dr R. A. McCall Smith. In their 1981 edition, and repeated in 1987, they identified eight situations, all of which are applicable to the sporting medical scene, which cannot be ignored by any medical practitioner, both generally and particularly in the present climate of spiralling aggressiveness of competition and risks in the playing of games at every level, from school age to senior citizenship. Thus, in *Affuto-Nartoy* v. *Clark & ILEA* (1984) *The Times*, 9 February, the defendant local school authority and its schoolteacher employee were held liable in negligence because an excessively enthusiastic games master innocently, and non-violently, tackled a smaller and less physically equipped pupil in a rugby game, with injurious consequences, and this principle was reiterated during preparation of this chapter with a similar decision by Leonard J in *Townsend* v. *Croydon Education Authority* (1989) *Daily Telegraph*, 13 April, p. 12. At the age of 14 the plaintiff had suffered a broken skull from an inadequately supervised playground 'kicking game' based on martial arts films. At the other end of the age scale, litigation is still pending between a retired golf-playing headmaster and a golf-playing opponent for an eye injury arising out of alleged negligence by playing a ball out of a bunker without sufficient warning. Such examples are sample illustrations of the extent to which sporting medical treatment can be required, extending beyond what was traditionally experienced by the average general medical practitioner before the sports explosion in a recreationally orientated society.

The following categories of negligence have been adapted from Mason and McCall Smith. Their application to the sporting scene can be summarised under each heading; but it should always be realised, adapting a judicial aphorism from the property world, that 'the categories of negligence are never closed':

1 Vicarious liability.
2 The reasonably skilful doctor; the usual practice; the custom test.
3 Misdiagnosis.
4 Negligence in treatment.
5 The problem of the novice.
6 Protecting the patient from himself/herself.
7 *Res ipsa loquitur.*
8 Injuries caused by drugs (*per se*, as distinct from the complex competition disciplinary issues already considered above).

Vicarious liability

Within this narrowly based chapter it is not necessary to consider the wider details of a superior's liability for another's wrongdoing within the scope of employment. This has long been established for hospitals, with the current administrative arrangements for apportionment of any damages awards between the various medical protection organisations and appropriate Government departments.* For present purposes, an ideal example of the principles applicable

*Since 1st January 1990 this has been superseded by National Health Service acceptance of damages liability within the service, but medical protection organisations and private insurance arrangements continue as before for liability outside the responsibility of the Health Authorities in England and Wales and Health Boards in Scotland and Northern Ireland.

to non-hospital and sporting medical malpractice emerges from the facts and awards by the British Columbia Court of Appeal. It upheld the trial judge's decision in favour of a claim by a 28-year-old professional ice-hockey player, Mike Robitaille, against his former employing hockey club, known as 'The Canucks' (*Robitaille* v. *Vancouver Ice Hockey Club Ltd* [1981] 3 DLR 288).

The Canucks club doctors and officials rejected continually sustained complaints of developing injuries suffered during play for the club. Negligence was proved because of what the court found to have been high-handed and arrogant forms of conduct, resulting in considerable loss and suffering. The doctors' legal nexus with the club to establish vicarious liability by the club comprised a relatively modest bonus of $2500: season tickets, free parking and access to the club lounge. The appeal court upheld the trial judge's evidential findings of fact that: 'The measure of control asserted by the defendant over the doctors in carrying out their work was substantial. The degree of control need not be complete in order to establish vicarious liability. In the case of a professional person, the absence of control and detection over the manner of doing the work is of little significance.' In support of this proposition the court cited an English court's decision in *Morren* v. *Swinton and Pendelbury Borough Council* [1965] 2 All ER 349.

Of equal importance for sports men and women was a concurrent approval by the appeal court of the trial judge's conclusion that the plaintiff was contributorily negligent. He was held to be 20% at fault because of his failure to take any action, i.e. to complain to protect his own interest, was less than reasonable. There was evidence upon which Esson J could find that Robitaille was negligent, '... the trial judge correctly distinguished cases ... which dealt with factory workers ... dealing here with a highly paid experienced modern day professional athlete and not a factory worker responding to the mores of olden times' 124 DLR (3rd) at p. 204.

In the context of a 'highly paid experienced modern day professional athlete', this judicial approach was reflected four years later by the English Court of Appeal in *Condon* v. *Basi* (see p. 71) when it ruled that in respect of the duty of care element in a claim for negligence based upon a foul tackle 'there will be a higher degree of care required of a player in a First Division football match than of a player in a local league football match.'

In Robitaille's case it is arguable that the plaintiff's contributory negligence assessment by the court for not pursuing his medical complaints to agencies outside the negligent club's control earlier than he did was possibly harsh. Nevertheless, the judge heard extensive oral evidence, and his final awards, which included aggravated and exemplary damages, demonstrated his ultimate awareness of the plaintiff's overriding and justifiable grievances of medical neglect which created a clear-cut liability. The awards at 1981 levels comprised:

1 $175 000 for loss of professional hockey income.
2 $85 000 for loss of future income other than from professional hockey.
3 $50 000 for the traditional pain, suffering and loss of enjoyment of life.

The principles applied here would certainly be operated in the UK courts. The reciprocity with which Commonwealth countries apply and extend the traditional Anglo-Saxon Common Law was ideally exemplified in *Condon* v. *Basi*. In that landmark decision, extending and applying the concept of negligence to a violent foul soccer tackle, the Court of Appeal in London adapted and applied the judgments of two Australian judicial sources, Barwick CJ and Kitton from *Rootes* v. *Shelton* [1986] ALR 33, a negligence claim for injuries suffered from a water-skiing accident.

ALR: Australian Argus Law Reports

Sports doctors should therefore recognise that, even without a formal contract, elements of access to a club lounge, free parking, season tickets and a modest $2500 bonus can create cumulatively a sufficient degree of control to place them and their associated club jointly at risk if negligence can be established.

Nearer home, two examples from the professional football world pin-point potential vicarious liabilities if the facts merit such a conclusion. One concerned the Swansea City and Tottenham Hotspur Company clubs. The other related to litigation between Queen's Park Rangers and Sheffield Wednesday.

The commencement of the 1956–7 soccer season coincided with the arrival at the Welsh club of a player, Derek King, who was signed for £2000 without having undergone a medical examination. The Swansea club's history, 1912–1982, explains how 'He played only five games at the Vetch Field before being forced to give up the game as a result of a knee defect ... the Swans claimed that King was unfit when he arrived, while the vendors held the opposite view. Unhappily for the Vetch men the contract was valid.'

The contractual terms were not identified, but the absence of any medical examination by a purchasing club would be unheard of today. Furthermore, if a club doctor were to misdiagnose an ascertainable medical flaw within the well-recognised medical legal criteria of Bolam's case (see p. 40) on an inspection before a transfer, and if within a reasonable time afterwards playing experiences should disclose such a medical flaw, the doctor personally could be at a substantial risk for any authentic loss suffered by the purchasing club, through loss of services or devaluation of the purchased player. Indeed, as these pages were being completed at the end of August 1989, a proposed £2 million pound transfer of Paul Ince from West Ham United to Manchester United was frustrated by an apparent discovery of a pelvic injury upon a medical inspection.

In 1977, Queen's Park Rangers failed to satisfy Judge Laughton Scott in the High Court that Sheffield Wednesday had misled the London club into paying £55000 for a player who had represented England's under-23 eleven, Vic Mobley, on the basis that his osteo-arthritic knee condition had not been disclosed at the time of the transfer transaction. After a 20-day trial, and a reserved judgment, which covered extensive medical evidence, the Judge concluded that Mobley disclosed no osteoarthritic symptoms at the time of the transfer. No appeal against the decision was lodged.

While these pages were being prepared, a graphic illustration of how vicarious liability can arise for sporting organisations emerged in dramatic form when under-21 representative England midfield player, Paul Lake, playing for Manchester City, 'swallowed his tongue' after a collision with an opponent in a Football League match. The club physiotherapist successfully remedied the condition and the Manchester City Club doctor, Norman Luft, highlighted the fact that immediate availability of medical attention was essential. He advocated the desirability of doctors being located near the touch-line in the conventional dug-out, rather than being remotely sited in the grandstand.

The Football League rules insist that a doctor should be present at the grounds during every game. The absence of a doctor could create an ultimate civil liability, coexistent with the absence of facilities, an area which the Sheffield Wednesday Hillsborough inquiry will investigate. Less renowned clubs will not be able to afford such professional assistance. Nevertheless, the absence of first-aid facilities at even the most humble of occasions could, in appropriate circumstances, create a liability on the club for compensation.*

A further example in this area emerged during the last few days before these pages were sent to the printers. During the course of playing on Saturday 11 November 1989 for Arsenal against Millwall the England international player David Rocastle endured a similar experience to Manchester City's Paul Lake, and again relief was achieved by the club physiotherapist. On this occasion the referee in accordance with usual practice had allowed play to continue without immediately having any reason to be aware of the extent of the injury. He was criticised unfairly by reason of this unawareness in not stopping play for medical attention, although in comparable circumstances such delay could be fatal. The Arsenal team doctor in

---

*The doctor's liability can only arise if he is put on notice of lack of facilities and equipment and then fails to explain to the club the necessity of their existence. With varying degrees of equipment and facilities a doctor appointed by any club should be under a continuing duty to alert that club of the need for elementary medical resources consistent with the club's finance, membership and crowd capacity.

attendance to the patient–player was Dr John Crane who has contributed Chapter 26. At p. 336 under the sub-heading of 'Prevention of injury' he explains: 'Managers, coaches and referees have an important part to play in the prevention of injuries.' This complements the opinions of Drs Adams, Wren and Whiteson (Chapter 18) for amateur and professional boxing referees and Mr F. T. Horan in Chapter 28 at p. 344 under the sub-heading of 'The management of injuries' for cricket umpires. To adapt a well-known legal maxim to this particular area of accident prevention and vicarious liability, it may well be said that the categories of potential liability for player care and damage limitation are never closed.

The need for vigilance and caution in diagnosis and treatment for varying circumstances, ranging from *ad hoc* and emergency situations at one end of the scale to normal consultantcy circumstances at the other, cannot be stressed too strongly, and leads on to the next category identified by Mason and McCall Smith.

The reasonably skilful doctor; the usual practice; the custom test

Lord Scarman and the House of Lords restated time-honoured general principles in two oft-cited pages. In *Sidaway* v. *Bethlem* (see p. 36) he referred to a jury direction by McNair J in the leading case of *Bolam* v. *Friern Hospital Management Committee* [1957] 2 All ER 118: 'As a rule a doctor is not negligent if he acts in accordance with a practice accepted at the time as proper by a responsible body of medical opinion, even though other doctors adopt a different practice. In short, the law imposes a duty of care but the standard of care is a matter of medical judgment.'

In *Maynard* v. *West Midlands Regional Health Authority* [1985] All ER 635, he extended this: 'I do not think that the words of the Lord President [Clyde] in *Hunter* v. *Hanly* [1955] SLT 213 at 217 can be bettered: "In the realm of diagnosis there is ample scope for genuine difference of opinion and one man clearly is not negligent merely because his conclusion differs from that of other professional men ... The tried test for establishing negligence in diagnosis or treatment on the part of the doctor is whether he has been proved to be guilty of failing to act as a doctor of ordinary skill would act with ordinary care."'

A valuable illustration of failure to meet the criteria of this section comes from Dr John Betts's contribution on 'Scuba-diving and its medical problems: the role of the doctor' when he refers (pp. 295–6) to 'the problems which may befall the unprepared casualty officer' when confronted with an insulin-dependent diabetic business executive whose 'apparent response to sugar was misinterpreted'. On a claim by the widow of the deceased victim, who had committed suicide, 'Very substantial damages were awarded against the Area Health Authority and casualty officer while the BSAC

SLT: Scots Law Times

CLYB: Current Law
Year Book
SJ: Solicitors Journal

and its members (who had accepted a dependent patient) were exonerated.'

A less satisfactory position for practical purposes is still on record from a first-instance judgment of nearly 40 years' antiquity in *Clarke* v. *Adams* (1950) CLYB 2707, 94 SJ 599. A physiotherapist's patient was warned when undergoing short-wave diathermy, 'When I turn on the machine I want you to experience a comfortable warmth and not anything more; if you do, I want you to tell me.' Expert evidence called from the Chartered Society of Physiotherapists confirmed that this was consistent with the normally prescribed practice. The patient did not report to the physiotherapist as requested that all was not well, and suffered burns. Slade J held that, having regard to the danger of burning to which the patient was being exposed, the warning given was inadequate and negligent. No appeal was lodged, but it is arguable whether a similar judgment would have resulted today.

Misdiagnosis

This category of potential liability is another where emergency pressures can extend the risk area. Mason and McCall Smith stake out the boundaries with the general comment: 'A mistake in diagnosis will not be considered negligent if the usual degree of dealings with patient's standards of care is observed but will be treated as one of the non-culpable and inevitable hazards of practice.' They also cited in a footnote a judicial observation: 'Unfortunate as it was that there was a wrong diagnosis, it was one of those misadventures, one of those chances, that life holds for people' (*Crinon* v. *Barnet Group Hospital Management Committee* (1959) *The Times*, 19 November).

Canada, however, again provides a direct example of liability which was established by the Ontario Court of Appeal. A 41-year-old tool and dye worker broke his right ankle when playing soccer with his son. A negligently erroneous X-ray prescription requiring attention to the right foot was compounded by a cascade of consequential errors involving several medical practitioners, including a radiologist, all of whom consolidated the earlier misdiagnosis. This resulted in the appellate court's confirmation of the trial judge's ruling that 'One negligent doctor could be liable for the additional loss caused by the other.' The appeal court also upheld the damages award of $50 000 for general damages, which included $34 465 for loss of income up to the date of trial (*Price* v. *Milawski* [1978] 82 DLR (3d) 130).

Dr John Betts's scuba-diving contribution also emphasises that 'the potential for mistaken diagnoses by both diver and doctor is large'; and this identifies a problem of communication which is as common to the lawyer seeking full factual foundation for a claim from a client, as to the doctor from his patient for treatment. It is also illustrated by Mr Richard Kendrick's contribution on 'Dental damage in contact sport: risk management for general dental practitioners' when he writes: 'Fractures of the cheek bone and mandible, however, show a much higher incidence in contact sports ... their diagnosis is important as further trauma before healing is complete can lead to marked displacement and complications ... important following a blow to the face or teeth that the appropriate X-rays should be taken to exclude such fractures. This may even apply after a blow to a tooth with no apparent loss of tooth substance. This emphasises the point that it is important to make a thorough examination of the patient who has been injured.'

Negligence in treatment

For this issue the formulae in the Sidaway case (see pp. 40–1) did not affect *Whitehouse* v. *Jordan* [1981] 1 All ER 267 when Lord Fraser explained at p. 281: 'The true position ... depends on the nature of the error. If it is one that would not have been made by a reasonably competent professional man professing to have the standard and type of skill that the defendant holds himself out as having, and acting with ordinary care, then it is negligence. If, on the other hand, it is an error that such a man, acting with ordinary care, might have made, then it is not negligence.'

With sports medicine evolving as a developing science and discipline with varying levels of experience for different sports and different parts of the anatomy and different ages and sexes, the possibilities of genuine conflicting and specialist opinions can easily exist. Speculation without real example cannot provide prophecy here. The legal formula has been laid down by the House of Lords in *Whitehouse* v. *Jordan* and is unaffected by the later opinions on Sidaway. Sports medicine must live with it until tested in the fire of evidentiary battles.

The problem of the novice

This issue is equally of concern to the club or organiser who does not provide for adequate facilities in accordance with conventional circumstance. The amateur club which permits an unqualified member to act as an *ad hoc* first-aid assistant without any professional experience, resulting in ultimate serious injury, is as much at risk as the hospital committee which is so unwise as to allow an inexperienced practitioner to carry out complex operations, usually reserved for mature and experienced staff. Thus a football club committee which employed an inadequate contractor to repair a grandstand, resulting in injury to spectators, was held personally responsible and liable in *Brown* v. *Lewis* [1986] 12 TLR 455.

Protecting the patient from himself/herself

The problem here is self-evident within the sporting scene; for instance excessively enthusiastic athletes striving to return to action when not fully fit or over-zealous coaches and team management committees, which are part of the recognisable pattern of command in every sporting discipline. Without firm medical guidance emphasising the harmful consequences of the zest for play overriding such medical advice, then a liability for negligence could well arise. The demands and stresses of competitive professional sport are particularly vulnerable in this category. Towards the end of 1988, a representative of Windsor Insurance Brokers Ltd, who act for the Football League and the FA explained, as recorded in the *Daily Mail*, 8 November 1988, that: 'Figures proved a third more players were forced out of the game than 10 years ago ... The risk of serious injury problems began to get greater after the 1966 World Cup. Films of some of those Bobby Charlton goals show how much space players had then. Nowadays, teams squeeze the game into so limited an area of the pitch that there is bound to be more physical contact. It's the pace the players are running that increases the risk of serious injury.' Correspondingly, Dr John Crane in his chapter 'Association Football: the team doctor' emphasises: 'It is inexcusable practice in the care of footballers to inject any sprained ligament with local anaesthetic and let him carry on playing. Such a practice will merely convert a minor injury into a potentially serious injury.'

Res ipsa loquitur

This penultimate stage in Mason and McCall Smith's classification of medical negligence is identifiable by vivid critical and literal judicial commentaries on it. In the House of Lords, Lord Shaw of Dunfermline commented in *Ballard* v. *North British Railway Co.* [1923] SC (HL) 43 qt 46: 'If that phrase had not been in Latin, nobody would have called it a principle ... The day for canonizing Latin phrases has gone past.'

SC (HL): Sessions Cases (House of Lords) (Scotland)

In a hospital negligence case Lord Denning as Denning LJ illuminated it with a judgment that the plaintiff before him on appeal was entitled to say: 'I went into hospital to be cured of two stiff fingers. I have come out with four stiff fingers and my hand is useless. That should not have happened if due care had been used. Explain it if you can' (*Cassidy* v. *Ministry of Health* [1951] 1 All ER 574 at 588).

Once again a Canadian precedent emphasises the point. The plaintiff entered hospital for treatment of a fractured ankle. He left with an amputated leg. No explanation existed. That evidence justified application of this principle with an inevitable judgment of negligence (*MacDonald* v. *York County Hospital Corporation* [1972] 28 DLR (3rd) 521).

Injuries caused by drugs

Laboratory developments, with their controversial conclusions evidenced by such publicised products as thalidomide and Opren, understandably led Mason and McCall Smith to comment:

> 'There is, first and foremost, a philosophical question as to the morality of providing an elaborate system of compensation for those who happen to be injured by drugs when others, who may have identical injuries caused by different factors, go uncompensated . . .
>
> 'From the point of view of the doctor or the pharmacist, the major concern over strict liability laws along EEC lines lies in the need to ensure that the manufacturer can be adequately identified in order to avoid claims being made against himself. This might entail elaborate bureaucratic procedures and the fear has been expressed that it could lead to further development of the practice of defensive medicine. An interesting American twist is shown in *Oskehbolt* v. *Lederle Laboratories* (1983) Or. 656 P.2d 293.'

Or. 656 P.2d: Pacific Reporter (Oregon, USA)

In the above-mentioned case, a doctor, having been successfully sued for prescribing a faulty drug, himself claimed against the manufacturers for negligently and fraudulently failing to warn physicians of possible harmful effects of prescription medicines.

From the point of view of the sports doctor, pharmacist and administrators, however, it is essential to emphasise once more: drug abuse and drug control within the world of sport demand special care from medical advisers. Any breach of that duty of care with risk of foreseeable damage or injury would create a prima-facie liability in negligence. They cannot now say that they have not been warned.

5. Sport's future for medicine and the law

The range of subjects covered in this volume demonstrates beyond doubt the interaction which exists between sports medicine and the law, for the benefit of sport and above all for the patients who are considered in respect of three areas: good health, education and self- or externally controlled discipline. The evidence from the medical profession and its associated activities ideally should form the guidelines for personal conduct and regulatory control. The control of cheating by drugs and violence is provided, not only by chemical testing in the former and referee control in the latter, but also by medical evidence which establishes the harmful and injurious consequences.

Public performance by athletes provides examples for future generations. This was confirmed by Alan Burns, the *Sunday Mirror*'s medical correspondent, in the issue of 16 April 1989. He cited the findings of the Institute for the Study of Children in Sport, where, according to its director, Martin Lee, a study carried out at Bedford College of Higher Education on 160 children disclosed that 'More than 33 per cent of ten year olds are prepared to commit a foul to gain an advantage', a percentage figure comparable to that disclosed by Davies and Gibson for injuries likely to be attributable to violent foul play resulting from their Guy's Hospital Athletics Injuries Clinic survey in 1978.

As the sporting scene and 'health and sport for all' campaigns expand yearly, sports medicine is well placed to monitor and steer developments for the benefit of society at large. Parliament gave a lead as long ago as 1970 when the Chronically Sick and Disabled Persons Act 1970 required public undertakings to provide access, parking and toilet facilities (including those relating to sport and recreation) which are practical and reasonable for a disabled person's needs. Section 5 of the Disabled Persons Act 1981 imposes duties on those who grant planning permission under Section 29 of the Town and Country Planning Act 1970 to draw attention to Section 4 and other provisions of that 1981 Act for the benefits required for the disabled.

At the time of writing in 1989 final conclusions are still awaited from the Home Office and Parliament on the 1987 proposals referred to on p. 29 for anabolic steroids to be added to the lists of proscribed drugs under the Misuse of Drugs Act 1971. Sporting bodies' regulatory powers are limited to their own discretion. Medical evidence for these particular substances' harmful consequences would impose more clearly identifiable sanctions on cheating athletes than the present sporting regulations can create.

The Hillsborough Sheffield Wednesday judicial inquiry will contain recommendations for promotional and organisational requirements. It is likely that they will reiterate and re-emphasise what has been on file and on record since earlier comparable inquiries — into Wembley Stadium crowd problems in 1923 (Cmnd. 2088 (1924)), Bolton Wanderers disaster in 1946 (Cmnd. 6846 (1947)), the Ibrox stand disaster (in 1971) and the Poppelwell Bradford City Fire Disaster Reports — which led to incomplete and limited legislation. Thus Parliament will fill the gaps on an *ad hoc* basis in the manner it has previously manifested when responding to sporting disaster.

Conclusions and summary

Every chapter in this volume demonstrates the need for special care in each sporting discipline. The requirements for boxers and jockeys are different in detail from the needs to protect cricketers, footballers and athletes. Nevertheless, the level of care by doctors, paramedical services, administrators and promoters and organisers must inevitably interact upon each other. Parliament's entry into these fields has been in the fragmentary manner identified here; and this echoes the prognosis recognised by the creator of the role of a Government minister with responsibility for sport, the former Lord Chancellor, Lord Hailsham of St Marylebone, when he was Minister for Science and Technology in Macmillan's Cabinet in the early 1960s. He foresaw a need: 'Not for a Ministry but for a focal point under a Minister for a coherent body of doctrine, perhaps even a philosophy of government encouragement. My eloquence had its effect on the Prime Minister and, before I knew where I was, I was left to organise the first government of this kind.'

In the intervening quarter of a century no holder of that post since then has held Cabinet office, and many different departments in Whitehall, Health and Social Security, Environment, the Home Office and Education, have fragmentarily been associated with the sporting health of the community. While need remains to protect communal health through the sporting scene, the one element which binds all sports will always be the role of medicine harnessed to the law at all its levels, playing, administrative and national. Therein lies the future well-being of sport and its role in the international community.

Appendix 5.1. The Central Council of Physical Recreation. Fair Play in Sport: a Charter

Introduction

Sport and physical recreation are generally recognised to be very important elements of healthy living and are primarily for the enjoyment and benefit of the participants. Organised team sports offer valuable lessons in social behaviour. They teach the importance of rules, the need to accept the decisions of officials, and the advantages of co-operation to achieve success. Young people learn by precept and example; they are influenced by the behaviour of their heroes in their favourite sports and by the attitudes of the reporting media.

Sport has been part of the social fabric in countries all over the world for a very long time. Growing prosperity, improved means of transport and the development of instant world-wide communications have brought about an explosion of sporting activity and spectator interest in recent years.

Many of the world's most popular sports and recreations had their origins in Britain, and many others owe their modern laws, structure and organisation to the pioneering work of British administrators. The value of concepts such as 'fair play', 'sportsmanship' and 'playing the game' are universally recognised, and are understood as the standard terms to express the idea that honourable conduct is an essential part of any sporting competition.

It must be sadly evident to anyone with a genuine love of sport that this traditional British approach to sport has undergone a radical change in recent years. It is widely felt that standards of behaviour and conduct among competitors, spectators and commentators have declined; harmful practices have crept in on a scale that threatens to undermine the very purpose of sport as a beneficial form of individual and social recreation. Even more worrying is the baleful effect on the younger generation of the frequent examples of serious misconduct and malpractice in many popular spectator sports.

The CCPR believes that there are many people who still passionately support the British concepts of good sportsmanship and fair play, who would like to see a concerted effort made to encourage a return to the standards that made British sport the envy of the world.

The laws and rules of sport are established by their governing bodies. The interpretation and application of the rules are in the hands of officials, umpires and referees; but the standards of conduct are set by the competitors and their coaches. Spectators, sponsors and promoters contribute financially and the media brings the sports to the attention of the wider public. The quality of every event is set by the standards of behaviour of each of these groups.

The following Charter calls attention to the urgent need for all the major participants in British sport — governing bodies, schools and clubs, coaches, competitors, sponsors, promoters and the media — to reaffirm the factors that constitute good conduct in sport and to strive for the highest ideals of sportsmanship.

Terms of the Charter

General

Members of governing bodies, officials, competitors and spectators are perceived by the general public as representative of their sports and must always attempt to set a good example, particularly to the younger generation, by the way in which they carry out their duties and responsibilities both on and off the field. The media plays a particularly vital role in this respect. It is urged, in keeping with the spirit of the Code of Practice agreed by Editors of national newspapers, to maintain the highest standards of responsible journalism in its reporting of sport and in its comments on sporting personalities.

Governing bodies

1 Must ensure that their rules are fair, thoroughly understood by competitors and officials, and properly enforced.
2 Must make every effort to ensure that the rules are applied consistently and with absolute impartiality.
3 Must make every effort to impress upon participants and officials the absolute need to maintain the highest standards of sportsmanship in the organisation and practice of their sport.

1 Must insist that competitors understand and abide by the principles of good sportsmanship.
2 Must not countenance the use of drugs by competitors.
3 Must never employ methods or practices that might involve risks to the long-term health or physical development of their charges.
4 Must not attempt to manipulate the rules to the advantage of their charges.

Competitors

1 Must abide by both the laws and the spirit of their sport.
2 Must accept the decisions of umpires and referees without question or protestation.
3 Must not cheat and in particular must not attempt to improve their performance by the use of drugs.
4 Must exercise self-control at all times.
5 Must accept success and failure, victory and defeat, with good grace and without excessive display of emotion.
6 Must treat their opponents and fellow participants with due respect at all times.

Sponsors and promoters

1 Must not seek improperly to influence the outcome of non-professional competitions by financial inducements.
2 Must understand and agree that the administration, operation and arrangements for the conduct of competitions and events are the exclusive responsibility of the governing bodies.

Conclusion

In order to bring about the raising of standards of behaviour across the wide spectrum of sport in Britain, the CCPR expects all governing bodies of sport and recreation, clubs, teachers, coaching organisations and spectators to give study to the Charter and take the necessary action to incorporate its relevant principles into their own rules and codes of practice and appeals to the Press Council to do the same.

Appendix 5.2. Extract from recommendations in the interim report on the inquiry of RT Hon Lord Justice Taylor into the Hillsborough Stadium disaster [presented to Parliament August 1989]

Co-ordination of emergency services

35 The police, fire and ambulance services should maintain through senior nominated officers regular liaison concerning crowd safety at each stadium.*
36 Before each match at a designated stadium, the police should ensure that the fire service and ambulance service are given full details about the

* These points were recommended to be carried out *before* the start of the 1989/90 soccer season. The rest of the recommendations in the report were recommended to be started forthwith and completed as soon as possible.

event, including its venue, its timing, the number of spectators expected, their likely routes of entry and exit, and any anticipated or potential difficulties concerning the control or movement of the crowd. Such details should be readily available in the control rooms of each of the emergency services.*

37 Contingency plans for the arrival at each designated stadium of emergency vehicles from all three services should be reviewed. They should include routes of access, rendezvous points, and accessibility within the ground itself.*

38 Police officers posted at the entrances to the ground should be briefed as to the contingency plans for the arrival of emergency services and should be informed when such services are called as to where and why they are required.*

First aid, medical facilities and ambulances

39 There should be at each stadium at each match at least one trained first aider per 1000 spectators. The club should have the responsibility for securing such attendance.*

40 There should be at each stadium one or more first aid rooms. The number of such rooms and the equipment to be maintained within them should be specified by the local authority after taking professional medical advice and should be made a requirement of any Safety Certificate.

41 The club should employ a medical practitioner to be present at each match and available to deal with any medical exigency at the ground. He should be trained and competent in advanced first aid. He should be present at the ground at least an hour before kick-off and should remain until half an hour after the end of the match. His whereabouts should be known to those in the police control room and he should be immediately contactable.*

42 At least one fully equipped ambulance from the appropriate ambulance authority should be in attendance at all matches with an expected crowd of 5000 or more.*

43 The number of ambulances to be in attendance for matches where larger crowds are expected should be specified by the local authority after consultation with the ambulance service and should be made a requirement of the Safety Certificate.

Epilogue

The number of contemporaneous occasions illuminating the subject throughout this text is indicative of the subject's developing potential. Three clear examples of this appear on pages 18, 24 and 47. During the time-lag between that cut-off date and the final date for proof corrections in mid-January 1990, the evolving pattern has not diminished. Football's world governing body, FIFA, banned Chile from the 1994 World Cup Competition and imposed severe sanctions on many of its medical advisers for falsifying medical reports about the condition of the national team goalkeeper and captain Roberto Rojas, who had feigned injury from a flare which had landed near him but did not strike him when the national team was losing 0–1 in a World Cup qualifying match against Brazil in Rio during September 1989. The English Football League announced its intention to appoint a supervising medical officer during 1990, and Lord Justice Taylor's anticipated *Final* Report will be required by protocol and precedent to be delivered to its commissioning Government Minister, the Home Secretary, who will decide upon its ultimate date for production after these pages have been finally corrected for publication. Furthermore, the Home Office is also the Government source dealing with prohibited drugs (and *not* the Department of the Environment which housed the Under-Secretary of State responsible for sport), which announced during early January 1990 that the Government intends to extend the Misuse of Drugs Act 1971 to make possession of muscle-enhancing anabolic steroids a criminal offence, two years after the Home Office announced in September 1987 its consideration for such an intention (pp. 29 and 46). As *The Times* recorded in a leading article on 29 December 1989, 'It has needed pressure from many quarters, particularly Mr Colin Moynihan, the Minister for Sport, and Mr Menzies Campbell, the Liberal Democrats' spokesman on sport, to put firmly en route to the statute book. They have done an important service'. Almost symbolically, a few weeks later in *The Times* Sports Letters pages for 11 January 1990 during a correspondence on the wider issue of British sport during the 1990s, the distinguished former international rugby referee and sports administrator, Air Vice-Marshal G. C. (Larry) Lamb, CB, CBE, AFC, explained the aim from his standpoint as General Secretary of the London Sports Medicine Institute in 'the closest consultation with the Sports Council, the BOA (British Olympic Association), BASM (British Association of Sports Medicine), and all other interested parties, including major governing bodies of sport, to translate this London orientated body into a national sports medicine institute serving the entire country.'

This target is consistent with what I have been increasingly aware of as the non-medical legal editor from my other editorial colleagues and sports doctors generally, namely the fragmented pattern of sports medicine throughout the UK. I had suspected this while I wrote the Introduction to my chapter 'Sports Medicine and the Law' in Butterworths' *Sport and the Law* (1988), without realising at the time that the concept had been first floated by Dr John O'Hara, Chairman of the Football Association Medical Committee. His initiative caused me to write then, 'The Football Association National Rehabilitation and Sports Injuries Centre has been opened at the National Sports Centre in Lilleshall, Shropshire; HRH The Princess Royal, as President of the British Olympic Medical Centre officiated at the opening of Northwick Park Hospital and Clinical Research Cantre in Harrow on the outskirts of North London; and London Sports Medicine Institute has been opened on the campus of St Bartholomew's Medical College. Yet Dr Dan Tunstall Pedoe, medical director of the Institute and medical adviser to the London Marathon explained to the *Daily Telegraph* (23 December 1986) "Sports Medicine has had virtually no official recognition or support from the health service. The average struggling athlete, let alone the serious amateur, is less well served here than in other countries, where there is government money for injuries and where there may well be well-established sports clinics."'

Throughout 1990, and beyond, successive Commonwealth Games and World Cup competitions in addition to countless other events will re-emphasize this justifiable complaint. Significantly, Larry Lamb's letter followed a three-part series in *The Times* assessing the world sports scene for the 1990s by Sebastian Coe and Daley Thompson in which they explained (5 January 1990) 'In many sports we still lose too many competitors too early through injury ... Ask any competitor what he or she most wants to see improved, and the answer will always be medical help.' I would extend that to anyone at *every* age and participatory level. Coe and Thompson claimed further, however, with words that could have been written intuitively with the following pages in mind.

> 'Doctors everywhere have to understand that they do not have all the answers. Sporting injuries require a multi-disciplinary approach. Often sports men and women need specialist insight and advice; for example, their reliance on a shoulder or knee is not that of most citizens. Few doctors have the knowledge and experience to treat every pull, strain, break or tear.
>
> 'Daley and I would like to see a national system in which specialists and interested doctors could co-operate effectively — aware of and able to call upon each other's help and guidance ... At any time, a wrong diagnosis, or treatment can ruin a career. Mistakes can never be wholly avoided. But what we need is an effective network, based perhaps on a central register, into which the best of our sporting talent (and their coaches and doctors) can plug themselves and get the best and the appropriate help when it is needed.'

If 'there is a tide in the affairs of men, Which, taken at the flood, leads on to fortune', then the pages which follow hereafter should provide a catalyst to cause the British Government to apply Lord Hailsham's general thoughts of the early 1960s of a need 'not for a Ministry, but for a focal point under a Minister for a coherent body of doctrine, perhaps even a philosophy of government encouragement', not only to the sporting scene in general, but to sports medicine in particular, for the general health and mental and spiritual health of the whole nation.

Uses and abuses of drugs in sport: the athlete's view 6

T. J. ANSTISS

'Better to hunt in the fields for health unbought than fee the Doctor for a nauseous draught'
John Dryden

Introduction

A knowledge of the relationships that exist between athletes and pharmacologically active compounds is of vital importance to the medical practitioner involved with athletes. Efficient prescribing can reduce both time off training and ameliorate the impact of illness on performance. The practitioner must also be aware of the fact that many athletes self-administer non-prescribed drugs in an attempt to improve their performance on the playing field or in the arena.

Prescribing for illness in athletes

Athletes are prone to suffer from the same cross-section of illnesses that may affect any other group or patients. In this respect they should be provided with the same treatment as anyone else attending their doctor. Care should be taken, however, with preparations likely to affect adversely the athlete's training (including their sleep and dietary habits), and also with drugs in any of the five classes banned by Olympic sports (see Appendix 6.1). The Sports Council will gladly advise where uncertainty exists.

It should be remembered that self-medication with certain over-the-counter preparations (most notably cough and cold remedies) can result in a failed urine test. It is the athlete's responsibility to know the rules and avoid such preparations,[*] as well as preparations about which he or she is uncertain. Ignorance of the rules is no defence. To prevent inadvertent ingestion of banned substances the Sports Council has produced a card the size of a credit card with information for athletes, and a more comprehensive list of permissable drugs (with their foreign names) for doctors (Appendix 6.2). However, if an athlete has an illness for which only a drug from the

---

[*] Professional advice sought by athletes on the subject of the admissibility of the use of non-proprietary preparations in sports does not fall under the provisions of the NHS. Such advice should therefore be sought on a 'private' basis and is subject to the common law standards for accuracy and competence.

90

Chapter 6
Uses and abuses
of drugs in sport:
the athlete's view

banned list will do, then a letter should be sent to the governing body of the athlete's sport informing them of the date of commencement and likely date of cessation of treatment. This is preferable to a letter sent after a positive urine test, which may be viewed with some suspicion by the powers that be.

Inflammatory problems

Most athletes in training are no strangers to musculo-skeletal inflammation, and a short course of aspirin (600 mg q.d.s.) is often of use in helping symptoms settle and expediting return to full training. Piroxicam may be the drug of choice, however (Heere 1988). The medical practitioner must take care to establish the athlete's current analgesic consumption, since many athletes will have self-medicated with over-the-counter non-steroidal anti-inflammatory drugs (NSAIDs), e.g. ibuprofen.

For musculo-skeletal inflammatory conditions which have not responded to an adequate trial of conservative therapy (i.e. rest, ice ultrasound, etc.) a local corticosteroid injection may prove effective. $1-2 \, cm^3$ of hydrocortisone acetate in 5% lignocaine is infiltrated into or around the affected region as appropriate using aseptic technique, and the area rested for 48 hours before commencement of a suitable rehabilitation programme (Roy & Irvine 1983).[*] Since local anaesthetics are one of the 'classes of drugs subject to certain restrictions', if an athlete is to have a local anaesthetic before or during a competition some sports require written submission of the diagnosis, dose and route of administration. The practice of prescribing parenteral corticosteroids to promote recovery from overtraining is not recommended.

Performance-enhancing substances

'We consider this [doping] to be the most shameful abuse of the Olympic ideal: we call for the life ban of offending athletes: we call for the life ban of coaches and the so-called doctors who administer this evil' (Sebastian Coe, Olympic Congress at Baden–Baden) (Donohue & Johnson 1986).

Brief history

The use of drugs for non-therapeutic purposes is both widespread and ancient. Man has cultivated vines, hemp, poppies, coca and tobacco plants to produce substances which alter perception and

---

[*] The risks associated with the procedure should be carefully explained to the athlete, and a record of this placed in the athletes notes. There is an increased risk of tendon rupture following repeated steroid injections.

mood for thousands of years, and has been seeking naturally occurring substances to improve psychomotor performance for centuries.

91

Chapter 6
Uses and abuses
of drugs in sport:
the athlete's view

South American Indians have used cocaine to decrease hunger and improve stamina on long marches and it is believed that West African peoples have used cola accuminata for similar purposes (Prokop 1970). It is thought that both third-century Greek athletes and the fierce Nordic Beserkers ingested psychotropic mushrooms prior to competition/combat (Prokop 1970, Todd 1987). So ingrained is the belief in the existence of such substances that modern mythology finds Popeye ingesting cans of spinach, and Asterisk impotent against the Romans without a draft from Getafix, the druid's brew.

More recently, in 1865, several swimmers in a canal race in Amsterdam were charged with taking performance-enhancing substances, and in 1869 cyclists were known to be using 'speedballs' of heroin and cocaine. Burk's (Todd 1987) claims that use of caffeine, alcohol, nitroglycerine, ethyl ether, strychnine and opium were common among athletes in the late nineteenth century, whilst French cyclists of the period are alleged to have used Vin Mariani (Murray 1983), a mixture of coca leaf extract and wine called the wine of athletes. Amphetamines replaced other stimulants in the competitive arena in the 1940s and 50s (though as late as 1956 at the Melbourne Olympics, doctors reported spasms in one competitor characteristic of strychnine poisoning), and anabolic steroid use is believed to have begun in the early 1960s. Testosterone and its esters became popular in the late 1970s, whilst growth hormone and human chorionic gonadotrophin have become the magic potions of the 1980s.

Current prevalence

Official estimates of the prevalence of drug taking are based on the failed urine test rate at major championships — usually about 2% of all samples. This is generally recognised to be a considerable underestimate resulting from sample bias, i.e. it represents only those athletes unlucky or stupid enough to get caught. Over 20 years ago, US Hammer-thrower George Fenn stated 'I cannot name one guy, and I know just about all of them, who is not using steroids'. Further evidence for the prevalence of such behaviour comes from an unofficial survey conducted at the 1972 Munich Games by Olympic discus thrower Jay Silvester (Silvester 1973). He sampled fellow athletes from seven nations and reported that 61% admitted using anabolic steroids in the six months prior to the Games. More recently, in the 1983 Pan-American games in Caracas, Venezuela, 19 athletes from ten different countries failed the dope test (Neff 1983). Twelve members of the US track-and-field team flew home after the announcement of the first positive results from the weight-lifting competition, and a large number of other competitors withdrew

92

Chapter 6
Uses and abuses
of drugs in sport:
the athlete's view

with sudden injury or performed well below standard, possibly to avoid being tested.

Doping control

Following the amphetamine-related deaths of several cyclists in the late 1960s, the International Olympic Committee (IOC) set up a medical commission charged with eradicating drug abuse in Olympic sports. Testing was first introduced in the Grenoble Games in the winter of 1968, and more comprehensively in the Mexico Games the following summer. The first Olympics in which testing for steroids took place was Montreal in 1976 after the development of a reliable radio-immunoassay technique by Professor Raymond Brooks, of St Thomas' Hospital, London. Six athletes were found to have traces of anabolic steroids in their urine at this festival. Testing at European track meets in 1979 caught several female athletes, including three of the world's top middle-distance runners. In 1982 the IOC Medical Commission added exogenous testosterone to its list of banned substances; testosterone abuse being deduced from an abnormal testosterone : epitestosterone ratio.

Various devices have been used by athletes and their aides to enable continued drug use without risk of disqualification. Traditionally the authorities have focussed their attention on attempts to detect traces of banned substances in the athletes urine at the time of competition. Athletes would switch to steroids with a more rapid excretion as the competition approaches, attempt to flush out the drug and/or use masking substances to effect excretion and make analysis more difficult. Athletes may also perform (or have performed for them) their own assay prior to departing for the competition, and then withdraw if found to be still excreting. Other techniques rumoured to have been used include the submission of clean samples from bottles left behind the cistern, from a bag in the axillae via fine tubing taped to the body all the way down to the meatus, or the allegedly stimulating but risky technique of 'urinary infusion' in which a close friend (if not before, then definitely afterwards) passes urine into the athlete's catheterised bladder.*†

Both the definition of doping and the list of banned substances have evolved over the years as athlete and chemist have tried to outwit each other.

Currently, doping may be defined as: '... the administration of, or the use by, a competing athlete of any substance foreign to the body, or of any physiological substance taken in abnormal

*'You've passed the dope test sir, but you are three months pregnant!'

†Doctors have a moral obligation to decline to be hired by any such athlete in these circumstances, there is no guarantee, however, that the unscrupulous technically qualified entrepreneur would not benefit from such a situation. Perhaps the answer lies with the legislators of the sports governing bodies to institute random year-round testing with severe penalties for offenders.

quantity* or taken by an abnormal route of entry into the body, with the sole intention of increasing in an artificial manner his performance in competition' (Donahue & Johnson 1986).

93
*Chapter 6
Uses and abuses
of drugs in sport:
the athlete's view*

The IOC bans five pharmacological classes of agents, three practices, and places restrictions on the use of three other classes of drugs.

Class A. Stimulants

These drugs — which include sympathomimetic amines and CNS stimulants — have proved popular with competitors in both endurance-based sports (e.g. cycling) and sports requiring explosive power and aggression (e.g. field events, weight-lifting, contact sports) due to their capacity to act simultaneously on the central and autonomic nervous system, musculo-skeletal system (improving muscular contractility) and metabolic systems (e.g. increasing the release of free fatty acids, FFAs). Their misuse has probably declined from a peak in the 1960s.

In Belgium in 1965, tests revealed that over 57% of professional and 23% of amateur cyclists were taking amphetamines, and in 1966 the first five competitors in the World Professional Road Race refused to take a doping test. One of the five (Jacques Anquetil) (Donahue & Johnson 1986) later said, 'everyone in cycling takes dope himself, and those who claim they don't are liars'. On the other side of the Atlantic, in a very different sport, the extent of amphetamine abuse in American football (and the adverse behavioural and psycho-social consequencies of such abuse) have been well documented by psychiatrist Arnold J. Mandell (1976) in his fascinating book of the same period *The Nightmare Season* and in a paper entitled 'The Sunday syndrome' (Mandell 1979).

The psychological effects sought by athletes from these substances include enhanced alertness and ability to concentrate, decreased sense of fatigue, elevation of mood, increased self-confidence and increased aggression. Undesirable effects include interference with timing in technical events (e.g. hammer-throwing, pole-vaulting), an increased risk of injury due to overconfidence and excessive aggression, unpredictable and potentially devastating psychological consequencies (e.g. schizophrenic-like psychosis) in vulnerable individuals, and death. It was the amphetamine-related death of 29-year-old British cyclist Tommy Simson during the televised climb in the 1967 Tour de France which contributed to the setting up of the IOC Medical Commission to eradicate drug abuse.

---

*This would include the use of 'blood doping or autologous transfusion, i.e. removal of a quantity of the athlete's blood in the 'training' phase for storage and replacement just prior to the event, producing temporary supranormal oxygen-carrying capacity of the blood.

94

*Chapter 6
Uses and abuses
of drugs in sport:
the athlete's view*

Class B. Narcotic analgesics[*]

The psychological effects of opium may have been known to the Sumerians, but the first accepted reference to poppy juice is in the writings of Theophrastus in the third century BC. In 1680 Thomas Sydenham wrote that 'amongst the remedies which it has pleased Almighty God to give to man to relieve his sufferings, none is so useful and efficacious as opium' (Goodman & Gilman 1985).

Nevertheless, these potent analgesics are banned by sports governing bodies to prevent athletes competing with the pain of injury masked: a situation which might lead to worse damage. They have little ergogenic potential, and are not heavily abused by the injury-free. The issue of pain relief to enable competition is dealt with in a later section.

Class C. Anabolic steroids

Biochemistry. 1771 saw John Hunter induce male characteristics in the hen by transplanting testes from the cock, and in 1849 Berthold demonstrated that the typical results of castration could be prevented by implanting gonads into castrated roosters. The belief that testicular failure was the cause of ageing in man led to attempts to isolate the active testicular principal, thought to be an elixir of life. Brown-Sequard claimed increased vigour and work capacity from a preparation in 1889, but it is unlikely that his aqueous extract had any significant quantity of hormone. Butenant obtained 15 mg of androstenedione from 15 000 l of male urine in 1930, and the active testicular prncipal itself was isolated shortly after. Elucidation of the chemical structure and synthesis of the hormone was achieved in 1935, to which the name testosterone was given (Goodman & Gilman 1985).

Originally developed for the treatment of patients with medical conditions, e.g. Fanconi's anaemia, hypogonadism or severe catabolic conditions, anabolic steroids are the result of structural manipulations of the testosterone molecule.[†] 17α-alkylation reduces first-pass metabolism and facilitates oral administration, whilst

---

[*] Not only are opiate drugs banned in the eyes of the IOC Medical Commission, they are also drugs which are illegal to possess in most parts of the world, unless prescribed or administered by a medical practitioner. In the UK controlled drug regulations apply. These drugs are of course invaluable therapeutic agents in conditions of severe pain, e.g. fractures. The practitioner should remember that if these drugs are administered to an athlete the clinical indication for treatment should be recorded as well as the type and amount of the drug given, in case the decision should later be challenged by the athlete, or the sport's governing body. A dose of opiate analgesic before or during an event effectively disqualfies the athlete from competition.

[†] Anabolic steroids are synthetically-produced compounds whose structure and function are similar to naturally produced male sex hormone by chemical manipulation. However, the molecule can be modified to make it have a longer-lasting effect and greater efficiency in stimulating protein (muscle) synthesis.

95

Chapter 6
Uses and abuses
of drugs in sport:
the athlete's view

esterification of the 17-hydroxyl group increases lipid solubility and permits depot administration. Both testosterone itself and its anabolic steroid derivatives may be esterified, with testosterone being available in proprionate, cyprionate and enanthate forms. Enzymic de-esterification leads to the slow release of the testosterone or steroid molecule, with the length of the ester chain determining the duration of action.

Androgens increase protein synthesis by both increasing the amount of mRNA produced by the cell nucleus, and by counteracting the inhibitory effect of cortisol on ribosomal protein synthesising activity. Athletes would like this effect to be limited to muscles, tendons and ligaments, but unfortunately (especially for female athletes) protein synthesis is also stimulated in other tissues — notably those associated with secondary sexual characteristics.

Nevertheless, anabolic steroids do differ in the relative balance of androgenic to anabolic effects they induce — this being measured by bioassay in 21-day-old castrated male rats. The effects of a sevenday period of steroid administration is assessed on the mass of both the levator ani muscle and the seminal vesicles, and this result expressed as a ratio; the 'therapeutic index'.

Regrettably, one still hears health professionals (and the British National Formulary) claiming that anabolic steroids do not provide advantages for athletes. Expressing such an opinion to individuals who know otherwise not only fails to change their behaviour, but also serves to reduce the credibility of medical opinion in their eyes. After sufficiently heavy training, athletes will often go into negative nitrogen balance. This is the result of stress-induced ACTH/cortisol release from the hypothalamic–pituitary axis. Since a major component of the action of anabolic steroids is to counteract the decrease in muscle ribosomal activity brought about by corticosteroids (Bullock *et al.* 1968) it is not surprising that these compounds will only benefit athletes training hard enough to go into negative nitrogen balance. The studies which failed to demonstrate improved training gains for subjects taking steroids generally failed to use sufficiently intense training and used non-specific methods for evaluation of strength (see Haupt & Rovere 1984 for an excellent review).

History of use. It has been suggested that members of the SS were given testosterone to increase their aggression (Silverman 1984). The earliest evidence of hormone abuse in a more sporting context comes from Dr John B. Zeigler (Todd 1983), the US team physician at the 1954 world weight-lifting championships in Vienna, who claimed that the Russian team doctor disclosed that some his team were on testosterone. A few lifters in the US then commenced this practice for themselves, switching to the anabolic steroid Dianabol (methandrosterone) when this was put on the market by Ciba-Giegy

96

Chapter 6
Uses and abuses
of drugs in sport:
the athlete's view

in the late 1950s. In 1962, Bob Hoffman of the York Barbell Club contributed a piece to *Health and Strength* magazine entitled 'The most important article I ever wrote' claiming tremendous gains for athletes using isometric strength training principles. He neglected to mention that several of them were also taking anabolic steroids, but when this became more widely known, anabolic steroid abuse began to spiral and isometrics went the way of the 'hula-hoop'.

Athletes had opened a pharmacological Pandora's box, and in many sports it became difficult to make the national team if you

Table 6.1 Adverse effects associated with anabolic steroid use

Hepatic
  Peliosis hepatis
  Hepatoma
  Cholestatic jaundice
  Elevated liver function tests

Endocrine
  Decreased luteinising hormone
  Decreased follicle stimulating hormone
  Decreased testosterone
  Testicular atrophy
  Acne
  Gynaecomastia
  Altered glucose tolerance
  Hyperinsulinism
  Decreased spermatogenesis
    Decreased motility
    Amorphous sperm
  Masculinisation in women
    Hoarsening of voice
    Hirsuitism
    Menstrual irregularities
    Enlarged clitoris
    Decreased breast size
    Alopecia

Cardiovascular
  Elevated blood pressure
  Increased low-density lipoprotein cholesterol
  Changes in triglyceride concentrations
  Fluid and water retention

Skeletal
  Epiphyseal closure

Subjective
  Aggressiveness
  Changes in libido
  Irritability
  Muscle spasm
  Nervous tension
  Headache
  Changes in hair growth
  Dizziness
  Nausea
  Euphoria
  Rash
  Changes in appetite
  Urethritis
  Scrotal pain
  Increased urine output

Originally published in Kibble M. & Ross M. (1987) Reprinted with permission from the American Society of Hospital pharmacists.

97
Chapter 6
Uses and abuses
of drugs in sport:
the athlete's view

remained drug free, let alone compete successfully in major championships. Drug testing on the day of competition did nothing to decrease drug use in the off-season, when steroids are of more use anyway in enabling more work to be done. Rumours abounded that drug testing was not always as random as it might have been, since officials and organisers were reluctant to catch big names who drew in the crowds. The 1977 statement of the American College of Sports Medicine (basically stating that these compounds were of no use to athletes, who must be mad to use them in view of the horrendous side-effects), drastically reduced the credibility of the medical profession in the eyes of many athletes who knew otherwise.

The increase in the prevalence and sophistication of drug testing, the hepatotoxicity of the orals and long half-life of injectable steroids led to a resurgence of interest in testosterone and its undetectable esters about ten years ago. There is speculation that this change led to increases in the rupture of biceps and quadraceps tendons resulting from either increased aggression, disproportionate strength gains compared to connective tissue hypertrophy, or a combination of the two.

Side-effects of steroids. Common and less common side-effects associated with anabolic steroid use are listed in Table 6.1. Users of these compounds sometimes claim that the dangerous side-effects have only been documented in already ill patients being treated with large doses of 17α-alkylated steroids for prolonged periods. However, there is a growing awareness of an association between sports-related steroid use and fatal and potentially fatal complications — notably, ischaemic heart disease and severe liver disease including tumours. Minor side-effects are exceedingly common, however, including virilisation in women. Psychological changes may be profound, including uncharacteristic violent behaviour and mood swings which may lead to strain and even break-up of marriages and relationships. A recent paper (Pope & Katz 1988) reports a frighteningly high frequency of psychotic episodes in regular users of anabolic steroids. A large retrospective study (JAMA 1987) is underway to examine for long-term adverse health consequences (especially in the cardiovascular and hepatic systems) amongst individuals who used steroids in the 1970s.

Steroid usage patterns.[*] Sophisticated patterns of drug taking have evolved in order to maximise gains, keep side-effects to a minimum

---

[*] This section has been included to provide an insight into the practices which are indulged by some athletes aspiring to the top level in their sport. To the medical practitioner who may have to treat the aftermath of this form of unsupervised self-medication the details and extent of abuse that can occur may be of technical interest. The authors and editorial board wish to emphasise that medication to enhance performance with banned drugs such as anabolic steroids is a practice which

98

Chapter 6
Uses and abuses
of drugs in sport:
the athlete's view

and beat the drug tests. Steroids are usually taken in *cycles* of between four and 12 weeks to enable endogenous testosterone levels and Liver Function Tests (LFTs) to return to normal between cycles. '*Stacking*' involves the taking of two drugs simultaneously — commonly an oral with an injectable (e.g. an Anavar/Deca-durabolin stack) whilst '*Shotgunning*' is the dubious practice of taking several preparations at once. '*Plateauing*' results from steroid receptor down-regulation, manifesting itself as failure to continue making gains at that dosage. '*Staggering*', or switching to a different steroid after plateauing on the first, attempts to combat this, but there is little evidence for its efficacy (unsurprisingly). *Human chorionic gonadotropin* (e.g. Profasi 5000) is used by some to expedite the return of endogenous serum testosterone levels to normal after stopping steroids (a kind of wake-up call for the testicles). Athletes on steroids will commonly switch to preparations with shorter half-lives (i.e. orals) as competition approaches, and may even be aware of their bodies clearance times (i.e. how long it takes for them to become 'clean'). The recent development of a test for exogenous testosterone administration (via testosterone : epitestosterone ratio estimation) may have led to some athletes administering testosterone/epitestosterone mixtures.

Supply. Athletes usually obtain their drugs from the black market, though steroids remain freely available over the counter in some countries (including, I understand, some EEC ones). Gymnasia form a major distribution point, where a word in the right ear and a few fivers can result in a selection of tablets, phials, syringes and bad advice. Mail order businesses exist, though not on the same scale as they do in North America (Taylor 1987), where a raid on a flat of a black marketeer uncovered over $2 million worth of steroids, including 3053 vials of Deca-durabolin, 84 vials of veterinary grade steroids and 2344 bottles of dianabol tablets. The athletic drug market is big business, as witnessed by the recent conviction of ex-British 400 m champion David Jenkins for running a drug smuggling enterprise in California.

Information sources. Athletes are commonly well aware of which preparations or combinations of steroids they do well on, and some keep meticulous records of dosages, training gains, mood changes

Continued from p. 95
is to be deplored on medical, ethical and philosophical grounds. The various regimes that are described are likely to increase the chances of serious side-effects. It is the view of the editorial board that doctors should take no part in providing any such drugs for these purposes. Furthermore, if pressurised or coerced into so doing they should report the matter to the relevant governing body of the sport concerned, whilst at the same time maintaining the anonymity of the individual 'patients' concerned.

99
*Chapter 6
Uses and abuses
of drugs in sport:
the athlete's view*

and side-effects, often going back several years. Other information comes via word of mouth from other users, coaches and health professionals* and from perusal of the medical and underground literature. One manual in the latter category provides a particularly useful insight into the attitudes of some of the hard-core steroid-taking fraternity. In it the authors review the latest drugs on the market, giving tablet data, availability, side-effects, black market price, etc. (a veritable *mims* for the gym). 'Straight facts' include: 'the more you take, the more you grow' 'the less toxic a steroid is for your liver, the less effective it is for growth', and 'there is no such thing as too much steroid'. There is no need to emphasise the dangers of such rubbish. Their advice on injecting is sound, however: 'if you insist on using anything larger than a 21 G for an injection, run your arm up the inside to make sure there aren't any mice living in it.'

Growth hormone. Growth hormone became popular in the late 1970s to early 1980s, due to the more rapid and more permanent gains it was alleged to produce in combination with its undetectability. Severe and permanent side-effects abound, however, including diabetes, acromegaly, arthritis and myopathy. Whilst the risk of Jakob–Creutzfeld disease has been eliminated with the development of biosynthetic forms of the hormone, early synthetic forms had an additional methionine group resulting in antibody formation in 30% of children treated (MacIntyre 1987). The long-term consequences of this are unknown.

Some athletes may attempt to increase the secretion of growth hormone from the pituitary gland by ingestion of certain drugs (including propranolol, vasopressin, clonidine and levodopa) or certain amino acids such as ornithine, arginine, lysine and tryptophan. The effectiveness of such methods is unknown, in marked distinction to the potential hazards.

Class D: Beta blockers[†]

The chronotropic action and peripheral reduction of physiological tremor produced by these drugs is thought to confer advantages

---

*The doctor's input into this situation must inevitably be negative, as there can be no justification for doctors to play any part in the provision of anabolic steroids for use in enhancing athletic performance. Any athlete seeking advice must be dissuaded and counselled regarding the risks attaching to this form of drug abuse (*vide infra*).

†There is little in the way of danger to health that can be attributed to the use of β_2-blockers, other than in overdosage. It may indeed be difficult to justify withholding these drugs where they are medically indicated, e.g. in a hypertensive patient, who takes part in a sport when the drug is banned, e.g. snooker. As always, a good medical history and examination well recorded, will distinguish the case where the drug is legitimately prescribed from that in which the competitor seeks to gain unfair advantage.

100

Chapter 6
Uses and abuses
of drugs in sport:
the athlete's view

in precision sports (Kruse 1986). Competitors in some of the more sedentary sports may require β-blockade for cardiovascular reasons, hence the governing bodies dilemma in separating those with *bona fide* therapeutic indications from the cheats.

Class E. Diuretics

Diuretics have long been abused by athletes in sports with weight restrictions (e.g. jockeys, wrestlers, weight-lifters) and also by body-builders to improve muscular definition ('cutting-up') before a competition. The potential for electrolyte disturbance is minimised by prudent rehydration and nutritional practices. Spironolactone may possibly have been used as an anti-androgen to decrease the virilising effects of androgens in women. Carbonic anhydrase inhibitors can supress or inhibit urinary excretion of sympathomimetics, and for this reason urine is pH tested in the initial screen.

Miscellaneous compounds

Probenicid (Benemid) is used to supress urinary excretion of certain drugs prior to competition (a 'masking' agent) and cyproheptadine hydrochloride (Periactin) may be used to increase appetite and facilitate weight-gaining. Thyroxine is sometimes used to assist weight loss, and ACTH may assist in recovery from overtraining and inflammatory problems. Dimethyl sulphoxide (DMSO), a carrying agent, was in vogue a few years ago as a panacea for all kinds of injury problems but seems to have fallen out of fashion. To increase further the risks associated with such drug-taking behaviour, they are commonly procured from the black market which is not renowned for its quality-control mechanisms.

Blood doping

The possibility of autologous transfusion (blood doping or blood packing) by athletes prior to competition came to the public attention during the 1972 Munich Olympics, when rumours circulated that the Finnish athlete Lasse Viren had used this technique to good effect. Mr Viren, however, attributed his 5000 m and 10 000 m victories to reindeer milk, and this author, for one, accepts this explanation. More recently, seven members of the US Olympic cycling team, including four gold medallists, admitted to having had pre-race transfusions (Gledhill 1982). There was a degree of coercion involved, with the coach hinting that those who would not agree might find their selection chances reduced. Further, instead of re-infusion of the athletes own previously venesected packed cells, in some cases this involved transfusion of whole blood from a relative, carried out in a hotel room close to the velodrome. So much for the Olympic Ideal.

The studies looking into the benefit to athletes of erythrocytaemia have, like the steroid studies, produced conflicting results (Buick *et al.* 1976, Gledhill 1982, Thomson *et al.* 1983). Again, this is likely to be the result of methodological shortcomings in the studies showing no effect. The theory behind the practice is that increasing the haemoglobin by transfusion will increase oxygen delivery to the working muscles and the capacity for aerobic work, providing that oxygen delivery is the limiting factor and cardiac output and blood distribution to the muscles is not adversely affected by the increased viscosity. Studies demonstrating no benefit (Gledhill 1982) have generally used inadequate re-infusion volumes and/or re-infused too early after withdrawal — before the body had replenished the loss. Also, the blood was more commonly refridgerated, which is known to result in greater erythrocyte loss than if it had been frozen. In summary, those studies which have shown improvements in aerobic capacity (Taylor 1987) appear much more likely to have induced an adequate erythrocytaemia.

Ethical issues

Is drug abuse by individuals engaged in sport so dangerous or immoral that those involved should be condemned? What grounds are there for so restricting an individual's liberty to do what he wants with his body?* John Stuart Mill strongly attacked any form of paternalistic restriction of individual liberty but only for fully autonomous adults. So one question to be asked is are drug taking athletes fully autonomous — or are they in some way coerced into drug taking? It is this author's experience that many athletes taking drugs would prefer not to, but since they suspect their rivals are drug-taking they feel that they must in order to compete without disadvantage. It is not considered cheating, just doing what everybody else does in order that the years of sacrifice and discipline are not all for nothing. Any reassurance to athletes that their rivals are not using drugs in the off-season would be a welcome development, and it is good to see that many sports are progressing down this road. Britain should be congratulated on implementing random off-season testing for its own athletes in advance of developments in other countries. The recent success of the British athletics team may partly be accounted for by a reduction in the chemically inflated per-

---

*The question of drug abuse in sport for the purpose of gaining unfair advantage presents a moral dilemma. The question facing the medical practitioner, society at large and sport in general, concerns the relative dangers that are presented by the use of powerful drugs in a non-therapeutic situation, when there exists because of them the possibility of damage to the individual through serious side-effects of the drugs, damage to the sport through the introduction of unfair competition, and damage to society at large through the erosion of its moral fabric.

101

Chapter 6
Uses and abuses
of drugs in sport:
the athlete's view

102

Chapter 6
Uses and abuses
of drugs in sport:
the athlete's view

formances of other nations, as more effective drug-testing strategies begin to bite.

Pain relief

What should the doctor do when asked to provide pain relief to enable an athlete to continue competition? There can be no hard and fast rules here, each situation requiring individual appraisal (Anstiss 1989). Factors to be considered include:

1 Is the injury likely to get worse if the pain is masked? (Broken nose or severe ankle sprain).

2 Does the athlete really want to continue, or is he or she being psychologically pressured by family, team mates or coach?

3 How important is the competition to the individual — is it his/her last chance for a British title, or just the street championships?

4 What other measures can be taken, e.g. equipment modification, changes in technique, protective taping?

5 Is the athlete intelligent enough to understand the risks and give informed consent?

6 Does the sport forbid or place restrictions on the contemplated practice?

For instance, if a 30-year-old wrestler in his final competitive year sustained a mild ankle sprain in the warm up prior to a major competition, and the resulting pain was obviously inhibiting his mobility, I would consider a local infiltration of anaesthetic followed by supportive taping, whereas I would not consider providing a similar service for, e.g. a young rugby player in an un-important game that his team was losing.

Steroid prescription

What should a general practitioner do if an individual enters his or her surgery requesting anabolic steroids by prescription, and/or regular monitoring of blood pressure and LFTs? Some physicians have argued that their wishes should be complied with, since the patient will otherwise take black market preparations of dubious quality. Arguments against this position abound, including the fact that athletes are unlikely to stick to the dosages prescribed, that such assistance might be interpreted as condoning the practice of drug-taking for performance enhancement, and that medico-legal consequences may result if recipients of prescribed steroids develop serious side-effects, as has happened in the USA (Thomson *et al.* 1983).

Such a consultation, however, provides an opportunity to assess the individual's knowledge and experience in the area, and disabuse him or her of any factually incorrect and possibly dangerous beliefs.

103
*Chapter 6
Uses and abuses
of drugs in sport:
the athlete's view*

Appendix 6.1: International Olympic Committee list of doping classes and methods

I. Doping classes

A Stimulants
B Narcotics
C Anabolic steroids
D Beta-blockers
E Diuretics
F Peptide hormones and analogues

II. Doping methods

A Blood doping
B Pharmacological, chemical and physical manipulation

III. Classes of drugs subject to certain restrictions

A Alcohol
B Marijuana
C Local anaesthetics
D Corticosteroids

Note

The doping definition of the IOC Medical Commission is based on the banning of pharmacological classes of agents. The definition has the advantage that also new drugs, some of which may be especially designed for doping purposes, are banned.

The following list represents examples of the different dope classes to illustrate the doping definition. Unless indicated, all substances belonging to the banned classes may not be used for medical treatment, even if they are not listed as examples. If substances of the banned classes are detected in the laboratory, the IOC Medical Commission will act. It should be noted that the presence of any drug in the urine constitutes an offence, irrespective of the route of administration (25 May 1989).

Examples and explanations

I. Doping classes

A. Stimulants

Amphetaminil	Benzphetamine
Amiphenazole	Caffeine*
Amphetamine	Cathine

104

Chapter 6
Uses and abuses
of drugs in sport:
the athlete's view

Chlorphentermine
Clobenzorex
Clorprenaline
Cocaine
Cropropamide
Crotetamide
Diethylpropion
Dimethylamphetamine
Ephedrine
Etafedrine
Ethamivan
Ethylamphetamine
Fencamfamin
Fenethylline
Fenproporex
Furfenorex
Meclofenoxate
Mefenorex

Methoxyphenamine
Methylamphetamine
Mehtylphenidate
Morazone
Nikethamide
Pemoline
Pentetrazol
Phendimetrazine
Phenmetrazine
Phentermine
Phenylpropanolamine
Pipradol
Prolintane
Propylhexedrine
Pyrovalerone
Strychnine
And related compounds

*For caffeine the definition of a positive depends on whether the concentration in urine exceeds 12 mg/ml.

Stimulants comprise various types of drugs which increase alertness, reduce fatigue and may increase competitiveness and hostility. Their use can also produce loss of judgement, which may lead to accidents to others in some sports. Amphetamine and related compounds have the most notorious reputation in producing problems in sport. Some deaths of sports men and women have resulted even when normal doses have been used under conditions of maximum physical activity. There is no medical justification for the use of 'amphetamines' in sport.

One group of stimulants is the sympathomimetic amines of which ephedrine is an example. In high doses, this type of compound produces mental stimulation and increased blood flow. Adverse effects include elevated blood pressure and headache, increased and irregular heart beat, anxiety and tremor. In lower doses they, e.g. ephedrine, pseudoephedrine, phenylpropanolamine, norpseudo-ephedrine, are often present in cold and hay fever preparations which can be purchased in pharmacies and sometimes from other retail outlets without the need of a medical prescription. *Thus no product for use in colds, flu or hay fever purchased by a competitor or given to him should be used without first checking with a doctor or pharmacist that the product does not contain a drug of the banned stimulants class.*

Beta-2 agonists. The choice of medication in the treatment of asthma and respiratory ailments has posed many problems. Some years ago, ephedrine and related substances were administered quite frequently. However, these substances are prohibited because they are classed in the category of 'sympathomimetic amines' and therefore considered as stimulants.

105
Chapter 6
Uses and abuses
of drugs in sport:
the athlete's view

The use of only the following β_2-agonists is permitted in the aerosol form:
Bitolterol
Orciprenaline
Rimiterol
Salbutamol
Terbutaline

B. Narcotic analgesics

Anileridine	Dipipanone
Buprenorphine	Methadone
Codeine	Morphine
Dextromoramide	Pentazocine
Dextropropoxyphene	Pethidine
Diamorphine (heroin)	Phenazocine
Dihydrocodeine	Trimeperidine
	And related compounds

The drugs related to this class, which are represented by morphine and its chemical and pharmacological analogues, act fairly specifically as analgesics for the management of moderate to severe pain. This description, however, by no means implies that their clinical effect is limited to the relief of trivial disabilities. Most of these drugs have major side-effects, including dose-related respiratory depression, and carry a high risk of physical and psychological dependence. There exists evidence indicating that narcotic analgesics have been and are abused in sports, and therefore and IOC Medical Commission has issued and maintained a ban on their use during the Olympic Games. The ban is also justified by international restrictions affecting the movement of these compounds and is in line with the regulations and recommendations of the World Health Organisation regarding narcotics.

Furthermore, it is felt that the treatment of slight to moderate pain can be effective using drugs — other than the narcotics — which have analgesic, anti-inflammatory and antipyretic actions. Such alternatives, which have been successfully used for the treatment of sports injuries, including anthranilic acid derivatives (such as mefenamic acid, floctafenine, glafenine, etc.), phenylalkanoic acid derivatives (such as diclofenac, ibuprofen, ketoprofen, naproxen, etc.) and compounds such as indomethacin and sulindac. The Medical Commission also reminds athletes and team doctors that aspirin and its newer derivatives (such as diflunisal) are not

106

Chapter 6
Uses and abuses
of drugs in sport:
the athlete's view

banned but some pharmaceutical preparations where aspirin is often associated with a banned drug such as codeine should be used with caution. The same precautions hold for cough and cold preparations which often contain drugs of the banned classes.

Dextromethorphan is not banned and may be used as an anti tussive. Diphenoxylate is also permitted.

C. Anabolic steroids

Bolasterone	Nandrolone
Boldenone	Norethandrolone
Chlordehydromethyltestosterone	Oxandrolone
Clostebol	Oxymesterone
Fluoxymesterone	Oxymetholone
Mesterolone	Stanozolol
Methandienone	Testosterone*
Methenolone	And related compounds
Methyltestosterone	

*For testosterone the definition of positive depends on the administration of testosterone or the use of any other manipulation having the result of increasing the ratio in urine of testosterone : epitestosterone to above 6.

This class of drugs includes chemicals which are related in structure and activity to the male hormone testosterone, which is also included in this banned class. They have been misused in sport, not only to attempt to increase the muscle bulk, strength and power when used with increased food intake, but also in lower doses and normal food intake to attempt to improve competitiveness.

Their use in teenagers who have not fully developed can result in stunting of growth by affecting growth at the ends of the long bones. Their use can produce psychological changes, liver damage and adversely affect the cardiovascular system. In males their use can reduce testicular size and sperm production; in females, their use can produce masculinisation, acne, development of male pattern hair growth and suppression of ovarian function and menstruction.

D. Beta-blockers

Acebutolol	Nadolol
Alprenolol	Oxprenolol
Atenolol	Propranolol
Labetalol	Sotalol
Metoprolol	And related compounds

The IOC Medical Commission has reviewed the therapeutic indications for the use of β-blocking drugs and noted that there is

107
Chapter 6
Uses and abuses
of drugs in sport:
the athlete's view

now a wide range of effective alternative preparations available in order to control hypertension, cardiac drug arrhythmias, angina pectoris and migraine. Due to the continued misuse of β-blockers in some sports where physical activity is of no or little importance, the IOC Medical Commission reserves the right to test those sports which it deems appropriate. These are unlikely to include endurance events which necessitate prolonged periods of high cardiac output and large stores of metabolic substrates in which β-blockers would severely decrease performance capacity.

E. Diuretics

Acetazolamide	Diclorphenamide
Amiloride	Ethacrynic acid
Bendrofluazide	Frusemide
Benzthiazide	Hydrochlorothiazide
Bumetanide	Spironolactone
Canrenone	Triamterine
Chlorthalidone	And related compounds

Diuretics have important therapeutic indications for the elimination of fluids from the tissues in certain pathological conditions. However, strict medical control is required.

Diuretics are sometimes misused by competitors for two main reasons, namely: to reduce weight quickly in sports where weight categories are involved and to reduce the concentration of drugs in urine by producing a more rapid excretion of urine to attempt to minimise detection of drug misuse. Rapid reduction of weight in sport cannot be justified medically. Health risks are involved in such misuse because of serious side-effects which might occur.

Furthermore, deliberate attempts to reduce weight artificially in order to compete in lower weight classes or to dilute urine constitute clear manipulations which are unacceptable on ethical grounds. Therefore, the IOC Medical Commission has decided to include diuretics on its list of banned classes of drugs.

NB: For sports involving weight classes, the IOC Medical Commission reserves the right to obtain urine samples from the competitor at the time of the weigh-in.

F. Peptide hormones and analogues

Chorionic gonadotrophin (HCG — human chorionic gonadotrophin). It is well known that the administration to males of human chorionic gonadotrophin and other compounds with related activity leads to an increased rate of production of endogenous androgenic steroids and is considered equivalent to the exogenous administration of testosterone.

108

Chapter 6
Uses and abuses
of drugs in sport:
the athlete's view

Corticotrophin (ACTH). Corticotrophin has been misused to increase the blood levels of endogenous corticosteroids notably to obtain the euphoric effect of corticosteroids. The application of corticotrophin is considered to be equivalent to the oral, intramuscular or intravenous application of corticosteroids. (See section IIID).

Growth hormone (HGH, somatotrophin). The misuse of growth hormone in sport is deemed to be unethical and dangerous because of various adverse effects, for example, allergic reactions, and acromegaly when applied in high doses.

All the respective releasing factors of the above-mentioned substances are also banned.

II. Methods

A. *Blood doping*

Blood transfusion is the intravenous administration of red blood cells or related blood products that contain red blood cells. Such products can be obtained from blood drawn from the same (autologous) or from a different (non-autologous) individual. The most common indications for red blood transfusion in conventional medical practice are acute blood loss and severe anaemia.

Blood doping is the administration of blood or related red blood products to an athlete other than for legitimate medical treatment. This procedure may be preceded by withdrawal of blood from the athlete who continues to train in this blood depleted state.

These procedures contravene the ethics of medicine and of sport. There are also risks involved in the transfusion of blood and related blood products. These include the development of allergic reactions (rash, fever, etc.) and acute haemolytic reaction with kidney damage if incorrectly typed blood is used, as well as delayed transfusion reaction resulting in fever and jaundice, transmission of infectious diseases (viral hepatitis and AIDS), overload of the circulation and metabolic shock.

Therefore the practice of blood doping in sport is banned by the IOC Medical Commission.

B. *Pharmacological, chemical and physical manipulation*

The IOC Medical Commission bans the use of substances and of methods which alter the integrity and validity of urine samples used in doping controls. Examples of banned methods are catheterisation, urine substitution and/or tampering, inhibition of renal excretion, e.g. by probenecid and related compounds.

109
Chapter 6
Uses and abuses
of drugs in sport:
the athlete's view

III. Classes of drugs subject to certain restrictions

A. Alcohol

Alcohol is not prohibited. However breath or blood alcohol levels may be determined at the request of an International Federation.

B. Marijuana

Marijuana is not prohibited. However, tests may be carried out at the request of an International Federation.

C. Local Anaesthetics

Injectable local anaesthetics are permitted under the following conditions:
1 that procaine, xylocaine, carbocaine, etc. are used but not cocaine;
2 only local or intra-articular injections may be administered;
3 only when medically justified (i.e. the details including diagnosis, dose and route of administration must be submitted immediately in writing to the IOC Medical Commission).

D. Corticosteroids

The naturally occurring and synthetic corticosteroids are mainly used as anti-inflammatory drugs which also relieve pain. They influence circulating concentrations of natural corticosteroids in the body. They produce euphoria and side-effects such that their medical use, except when used topically, requires medical control.

Since 1975, the IOC Medical Commission has attempted to restrict their use during the Olympic Games by requiring a declaration by the team doctors, because it was known that corticosteroids were being used non-therapeutically by the oral, intramuscular and even the intravenous route in some sports. However, the problem was not solved by these restrictions and therefore stronger measures designed not to interfere with the appropriate medical use of these compounds became necessary.

The use of corticosteroids is banned except for topical use (aural, opthalmological and dermatological), inhalational therapy (asthma, allergic rhinitis) and local or intra-articular injections.

Any team doctor wishing to administer corticosteroids intra-articularly or locally to a competitor must give written notification to the IOC Medical Commission.

110

Chapter 6
Uses and abuses
of drugs in sport:
the athlete's view

Appendix 6.2: Information for athletes, coaches and medical practitioners on the permissible use of drugs in amateur sport

(From the IOC Medical Commission)

Introduction (please read this section carefully before using this guide)

The only legitimate use of drugs in sports is under the supervision of a physician for a clinically justified purpose. The International Olympic Committee (IOC) and international sports organizations initiated drug testing to protect amateur athletes from the potential unfair advantage that might be gained by those athletes who take drugs in an attempt to increase performance. Drug testing is also meant as deterrent to protect athletes from the potential harmful side-effects which some drugs can produce.

The list of banned drugs contains a very small percentage of the currently available pharmacological arsenal and does not hinder the proper treatment of athletes for justifiable therapeutic reasons.

The following list of *permitted classes of drugs* is offered to the international sports community as a guide only. It is not comprehensive. Part I is a partial compilation which gives examples of drugs and preparations widely used in some countries or on some continents. Part II lists the generic names of corresponding drugs.

The list covers a number of therapeutic and/or pharmacological classes which are considered to be the most useful and which are used in the treatment of some ailments fairly common in those individuals who practice sport. The IOC Medical Commission wishes to state that the inclusion of brand names does not constitute in anyway an endorsement of the product nor a recommendation of the efficacy of the various substances these products contain. Furthermore, the absence of a product from the list does not constitute an unfavourable judgment, on the part of the Medical Commission, nor a recommendation against its use. Again, the list is provided for information purposes only.

The list mainly comprises drugs available on prescription from a medical doctor. It should be realized that a number of preparations containing banned drugs are available, from pharmacies in many countries, without a prescription. Care should be exercised particularly when obtaining treatment for pain, colds, headaches and nasal and bronchial problems. Likewise, preparations containing only an antibiotic or an antihistamine are permissible. However, care should be taken not to use an antihistamine tablet or liquid preparation which contains ephedrine or another sympathomimetic amine.

Very often, the same brand name covers different preparations, one or many of which may contain a banned drug. Some vitamin

111

Chapter 6
Uses and abuses
of drugs in sport:
the athlete's view

preparations sold in some countries also contain banned drugs such as psychomotor stimulants or anabolic steroids. Also remember that the rules of some International Federations may not allow the use of certain substances (such as tranquillisers) which are permitted in some sports. The IOC Medical Commission encourages individual countries to use this guide for establishing their own list of permissible drugs.

The IOC Medical Commission invites all those involved in sports to be cautious with drugs. During the Olympic Games, more information may be obtained from the Medical Commission by leaving a message in a specially identified box in the Olympic Village.

Part I

1. Antacids and some other gastrointestinal agents like anti-diarrhoeals

Acinorm (DEN), Alcap (ITA), Aldrox, (ARG), Alka-2 (USA), Allulose (NOR), Altacit (GBR), Aludrox (GBR), Alumag (S.AFRI), Aluminox (HOL), Amphojel (ARG, CAN, S. AFRI), Andursil (GBR), Antepsin (GBR, ARG, ITA), Cantil (AUS, CAN, FRA, USA), Colofac (AUS, GBR), Diarsed (FRA), Diloran (GBR), Diovol (GBR), Donnagel (CAN), Duspatal (FRG, HOL, ITA), Equilet (USA), Gamma-gel (ITA), Gastridine (ARG), Gaviscon (AUS, GBR), Gelusil (CAN, GBR), Hi-Ti (JPN), Imodium (AUS, BEL, CAN, DEN, FRA, FRG, GBR, HOL, ITA, S.AFRI, SUI, USA), Kaomycin (GBR), Kaopectate (GBR), Lomotil (AUS, CAN, S. AFRI, USA), Maalox (GBR, CAN), Milid (FRG, ITA, S.AFRI, SUI), Nacid (JPN), Palmicol (FRG), Pepto-Bismol (GBR), Prodexin (GBR), Promid (JPN), Reasec (ITA, SUI), Rinveral (ESP), Riopan (CAN, ITA, FRG, USA), Riopone (S.AFRI), Robalate (CAN, USA), Sulcrate (CAN), Talcid (FRG), Titralac (GBR), Tralanta (JPN), Ulcerban (USA), Ulcermin (JPN), Ulsanic (S.AFRI), Unigest (GBR).

Beware

Do not take preparations containing codeine or opium e.g. Diban, Donnagel-PG capsules.

2. Anti-asthmatic agents and anti-allergenic agents

*Albuterol (USA), Aldecin (AUS, BEL, GBR, JAP, SUI, SWE), *Alotec (JPN), *Alupent (ARG, CAN, FRG, S.AFRI), Aminodur (USA), Asmafil (ITA), *Asmaten (ARG), *Asmatol (ARG), *Asmidon (JPN), *Astmopent (POL), *Astop (ISR), Atrovent (AUS, BEL, FRG, HOL,

112

*Chapter 6
Uses and abuses
of drugs in sport:
the athlete's view*

SUI, SWE), Beclovent (CAN, USA), *Beconase (AUS, BEL, CAN, FRG, GBR, HOL, SUI), *Becotide (AUS, BEL, CAN, ESP, GBR, JAP, NOR, S.AFRI, SUI, SWE), *Bitolterol mesylate (USA), *Bricalin (ISR), *Bricanyl (ARG, FRG, GBR, SWE, S.AFRI), *Bristurin (JPN), Bronkodyl (USA), Cardophyllin (AUS), Choledyl (AUS, CAN, DEN, S.AFRI, USA), Corophyllin (CAN), *Dosalupent (ITA), Euphyllin (FRG, S.AFRI), Euspirax (FRG), *Feevone (AUS), Intal (ARG, AUS, CAN, ESP, FRG, GBR, JAP, SUI, USA), Lomisdal (BEL, DEN, FRA, HOL, ITA, S.AFRI, SUI, SWE), *Metaprel (USA), *Pulmadil (AUS, BEL, DEN, S.AFRI), *Salbutan (ITA), *Salbutol (TUR), *Sultanol (FRG, JPN), *Terbasmin (ITA), Theocoline (JPN), Theo-Dur (CAN), Theolair (BEL, CAN, HOL, SWE), Theovent (USA), *Ventolin (ARG, CAN, ITA, S.AFRI, USA).

*Beware

These β-agonists are permitted in aerosol (inhalation form) only. Refer to the IOC list of banned classes and methods for restrictions regarding these drugs and the use of corticosteroids for the treatment of asthma.

3. Anti-nauseants and anti-emetic agents

Anaus (ITA), Antivert (USA), Aviomarine (POL), Bonamine (CAN), Dramamine (AUS, BEL, CAN, ESP, FRA, FRG, HOL, S.AFRI, USA), Emetrol (CAN), Gravol (CAN, GBR), Ibikin (ITA), Maxolon (AUS, BEL, FRA, S.AFRI, SUI), Neptusan (DEN), Nibromin-A (JPN), Postafen (DEN, HOL, NOR), Primperan (AUS, BEL, FRA, S.AFRI, SUI), Reglan (CAN), Scop (transdermal) (AUS), Stemetil (CAN), Tigan (USA), Torecan (ARG, CAN, FRA, FRG, ITA, USA), Transderm (CAN), Vertigon (GBR), Vomex A (FRG), Yesdol (JPN), Yophadol (JPN).

4. Anti-ulcer drugs

Biogastrone (AUS, BEL, CAN, FRG, GBR, HOL, JAP, S.AFRI, SUI), Burimamide (GBR), Cimetum (ARG), Gastromet (ITA), Metiamide (GBR), Metoclol (JPN), Primperan (AUS, BEL, DEN, FRA, GBR, HOL, NOR, S.AFRI, SUI), Reglan (CAN, USA), Tagamet (ARG, BEL, CAN, ESP, FRA, FRG), Zantac (GBR).

5. Aspirin and similar analgesic (non-narcotic) and anti-inflammatory non-steroidal agents

Acetamol (ITA), Acetard (DEN, SWE), Acetylin (FRG), Adiro (ARG, BEL, HOL, ESP), Alcacyl (SUI), Allopydin (JPN), Aluprin (USA),

113
Chapter 6
Uses and abuses
of drugs in sport:
the athlete's view

Anaprox (USA), Aquaprin (S.AFRI), Arlef (AUS, BEL, FRA, FRG, ITA, S.AFRI, SUI), Asatard (ITA), Aspasol (S.AFRI), Aspirin, Benortan (BEL, DEN, FRA, FRG, HOL, SUI), Benotabol (ARG), Ben-U-Ron (BEL, FRG, SUI), Bonabol (JPN), Brufen (AUS, BEL, DEN, FRG, JPN, S.AFRI), Bufemid (BRA), Calip (ARG), Capisten (JPN), Cinnamin (JPN), Cinopal (ITA, S.AFRI, SUI), Clinoril (ARG, AUS, BEL, CAN, DEN, GBR, ITA, HOL, S.AFRI, SUI, USA), Cresopirine (FRA), Desinflam (ARG), Dirox (ARG), Dispril (BEL, NOR, SWE, SUI), Dolisal (PER), Dolobid (AUS, GBR, ITA), Dorbid (BRA), Droxaryl (BEL, HOL), Ecotrin (AUS, CAN, USA), Ennagesic (S.AFRI), Enteretas (ARG), Entrophen (CAN), Enzamin (JPN), Feldene (GBR), Flanax (BRA, MEX), Flosint (ARG, ITA, S.AFRI), Glifanan (ARG, BEL, FRA, HOL, FRG, ESP, S.AFRI, SUI), Hyprin (JPN), Idarac (ARG, BEL, CAN, FRA, ITA, S.AFRI), Imotryl (FRA), Indacin (JPN), Indocid (ARG, AUS, BEL, CAN, DEN, FRA, ITA, S.AFRI, SUI, USA), Istopirine (HUN), Motrin (CAN, USA), Naixan (JPN), Nalfon (DEN, ESP, SUI, USA), Naprosyn (ARG, AUS, CAN, DEN, GBR, FRG, S.AFRI, USA), Norfemac (CAN), Orudis (CAN, DEN, ITA, JPN, ESP, S.AFRI), Paloxin (S.AFRI), Panadol (AUS, GBR, FIN), Paramidin (JPN), Pasalin (JPN), Pentosol (ESP), Ponstan (AUS, CAN, BEL, GBR, S.AFRI, SUI), Ponstel (USA), Pontal (JPN), Prinalgin (S.AFRI), Profenid (ARG, FRA, SUI), Progesic (GBR), Prolix (S.AFRI), Prolixan (BELG, DEN, FRA, FRG, HUN, ITA, HOL, SUI), Rheumox (GBR), Rhonal (ARG, BEL, CAN, JAP, HOL, S.AFRI), Salitison (JPN), Sedalgin (AUS), Sedapyren (S.AFRI), Sulindac (GBR), Superpyrin (TCH), Tamas (ARG), Tandearil (CAN, SUI), Tanderil (ARG, AUS, BEL, DEN, FRA, FRG, ITA, HOL, ESP, S.AFRI, SUI), Tantum (ARG, AUS, DEN, FRG, HOL, ITA, S.AFRI), Tolectin (BEL, CAN, DEN, FRG, S.AFRI), Tylenol (BEL, CAN, SUI, USA), Voltaren (ARG, BEL, DEN, FRG, ITA, JPN, ESP, SUI), Winolate (S.AFRI), Zubirol (ARG), Zumaril (ITA).

Beware

Do not take preparations containing codeine, morphine, heroin, opium, ephedrine.

6. Contraceptives

Anacyclin (FRG, SUI), Brevinor (AUS, GBR, S.AFRI), Conova 30 (GBR), Demulen 50 (CAN, GBR, S.AFRI, SWE, USA), Eugynon (ARG, BEL, DEN, FRG, GBR, HOL, ITA, NOR, SUI), Exluton (ARG, BEL, FRA, HOL, S.AFRI), Femulen (GBR, S.AFRI), Micronovum (FRG, S.AFRI, SUI), Minilyn (GBR), Nordiol (ARG, AUS, S.AFRI), Ortho-novum (AUS, BEL, CAN, FRG, HOL, ITA, SUI, USA), Ovostat (BEL, HOL, SUI), Ovral (ARG, CAN, S.AFRI, USA), Ovulen (ARG, AUS, ESP, FRA, FRG, HOL, GBR, SUI, USA).

114

*Chapter 6
Uses and abuses
of drugs in sport:
the athlete's view*

7. Decongestants and nasal preparations

Afrazine (GBR), Beconase (AUS, BEL, CAN, FRG, GBR, HOL, S. AFRI, SUI), Iliadin (GBR, FRA, S.AFRI), Lidil (ARG), Nafrine (CAN), Naphazoline HCl (ARG, AUS, BEL, BRA, JPN, USA), Nasivin (FRG, ITA, HOL), Otrivin(e) (AUS, BEL, CAN, DEN, ITA, HOL, NOR, S.AFRI, SUI, USA), Rynacrom (AUS, BEL, HOL, S.AFRI), Soframycin (BEL, FRA, GBR), Tyzine (AUS, BEL, DEN, ESP, FRG, S.AFRI, SUI, USA).

Beware

Do not use preparations containing 'sympathomimetic amines' such as pseudoephedrine, phenylpropanolamine, etc.

8. Expectorants and cough suppressants

Syrups: Balminil DM (CAN), Bisolvon (AUS, BEL, DEN, FRG, GBR, HOL, ITA, JAP, LUX, NOR, S.AFRI, SWE, SUI), Cosylan (GBR), Dextphan (JPN), Muflin (GBR), Reorganin (FRG), Resyl (BEL, CAN, ESP, SWE, SUI), Robitussin plain (AUS, CAN, GBR, ITA), Sancos (GBR).

Tablets: Astomin (JPN), Bisolvon (AUS, BEL, DEN, FRG, GBR, HOL, ITA, JAP, LUX, NOR, S.AFRI, SWE, SUI), Bractos (ARG), Hustazol (JPN), Lysobex (ITA), Respirex (ESP), Sinecod (BEL, FRG, ESP, ITA, SUI), Tessalon (CAN, NOR, SWE, SUI, USA), Tessalin (NOR).

Lozenges: Balminil pastilles (CAN), Bradosol (CAN, DEN), Cepacol (AUS, CAN, USA), Coricidin throat lozenges (CAN), Merocets (GBR), Neo-Bradoral (SUI).

Suppositories: Demo-Cineol (CAN), Medicil (ITA), Plausitin (ARG, ITA).

Beware

Most cough syrups contain one or several banned drugs.

9. Griseofulvin and other antifungal agents

Ancotil (ARG, AUS, CAN, DEN, FRA, FRG, JPN, NOR, SWE, SUI), Batrafen (BRA, JPN), Canesten (AUS, CAN, DEN, FRG, GBR, HOL, ESP, ITA, NOR, S.AFRI, SUI, SWE), Empecid (ARG, JPN), Eparol

(FRG), Fasign (ARG, AUS, GEL, DEN, HOL, NOR, S.AFRI, SUI, SWE), Fulcin (FRA), Fulvicin (CAN, USA), Fungilin (AUS, DEN, GBR, ITA), Fungo-Polycid (ESP), Grisovin(e) (AUS, GBR, AFR, SUI, SWE), Monistat (CAN, GBR, SUI, USA), Mycostatin (ARG, AUS, CAN, DEN, FRA, ITA, NOR, ESP, S.AFRI, SUI, USA), Pimafucin (AUS, BEL, FRG, GBR, ITA, NOR, S.AFRI, SUI), Tinactin (CAN, SUI, USA), Tinaderm (ARG, AUS, GBR, ESP, ITA, S.AFRI).

10. Haemorrhoidal preparations

Anucaine (GBR), Anusol (GBR), Cinkain (DEN, SWE), Nestosyl (GBR), Nupercainal (BEL, CAN, DEN, ITA, SUI, USA).

Beware

Some anti-haemorrhoidal preparations contain hydrocortisone. See the IOC list of banned classes and methods regarding the use of corticosteroids.

11. Hypnotics, sedatives and tranquillisers

Abasin (FRG), Adalin (FRG, HOL), Amytal (AUS, BEL, CAN, HOL, ITA, USA), Ativan, (AUS, CAN, GBR, S.AFRI, USA), Benzolani (URS), Brovarin (JPN), Chloralol (CAN), Dalmadorm (FRG, HOL, NOR, AFR, ITA, SUI), Dalmane (AUS, CAN, GBR, USA), Dalmate (JPN), Doriden(e) (BEL, CAN, DEN, ITA, USA, GBR), Dormogen (TCH), Equanil (AUS, CAN, DEN, FRA, GBR, S.AFRI, USA), Euhypnos (AUS, GBR), Evidorm (GBR), Evipan (FRG), Gardenal (BEL, CAN, FRA, ITA, ESP, S.AFRI), Halcion (BEL, CAN, DEN, GBR, S.AFRI, SUI), Haldol (BEL, CAN, FRA, FGR, GBR, SUI, SWE, USA), Largactil (AUS, BEL, CAN, DEN, ESP, FRA, GBR, HOL, ITA, NOR, S.AFRI, SUI), Levanxol (BEL, ESP, HOL, S.AFRI), Lexotan (AUS, BEL, DEN, ITA, JPN, S.AFRI), Librium (AUS, BEL, CAN, DEN, FRA, FRG, GBR, HOL, ITA, NOR, S.AFRI, SUI, USA), Mebaral (CAN, USA), Medomin (CAN, FRG, GBR, HOL, SUI), Mogadon (ARG, AUS, BEL, DEN, FRA, FRG, GBR, ITA, NOR, S.AFRI, SUI), Nembutal (AUS, BEL, DEN, FRA, FRG, GBR, HOL, ITA, SUI, USA), Noludar (BEL, CAN, DEN, FRG, GBR, S.AFRI, SUI, USA), Noctec (AUS, CAN, GBR, USA), Normison (AUS, GBR, S.AFRI), Prominal (AUS, BEL, GBR, ESP, ITA), Restoril (CAN, USA), Restwel (S.AFRI), Schlafen (JPN), Serenid (GBR), Serepax (AUS), Sobile (ESP), Soneryl (AUS, BEL, CAN, DEN, FRA, HOL, S.AFRI, SUI), Sopental (S.AFRI), Stelazine (AUS, CAN, GBR, S.AFRI, USA), Theobromine (—), Tranxene (AUS, BEL, CAN, FRA, GBR, HOL, NZL, S.AFRI, USA), Tuinal (GBR, CAN, USA), Valamin (FRG), Vallium (ARG, AUS, BEL, CAN, DEN, FRA, FRG, GBR, HOL, ITA, NOR, S.AFRI, SUI, USA).

115
Chapter 6
Uses and abuses
of drugs in sport:
the athlete's view

116

Chapter 6
Uses and abuses
of drugs in sport:
the athlete's view

12. *Insulin and other antidiabetic agents*

Daonil (ALG, ARG, AUS, BEL, DEN, FRA, HOL, ITA, NOR, S.AFRI, TUN), Diaben (ARG), Diabinese (ARG, AUS, BEL, CAN, GBR, HOL, ITA, NOR, S.AFRI, USA), Diamicron (AUS, FRA, GBR, ITA, S.AFRI), Dibotin (GBR), Dimelor (ARG, AUS, BEL, CAN, GBR, ITA, S.AFRI), Dipar (ESP, S.AFRI), Gilemal (HUN), Glucophage (AUS, BEL, CAN, DEN, FRA, FRG, HOL, ITA, NOR, S.AFRI, SUI, SWE), Gludease (JPN), Glutril (DEN, FRA, FRG, GBR, S.AFRI, SWE, SUI), Insoral (AUS, S.AFRI), Insulin (—), Islotin (ARG), Nadisan (ARG, BEL, FRG, ESP, SWE, SUI), Nigloid (JPN), Nogluc (ARG), Ordimel (HOL, SWE), Orinase (CAN, USA), Promide (AUS), Rastinon (AUS, BEL, DEN, GBR, ITA, NOR, S.AFRI, SUI), Silubin Retard (BEL, ESP, S.AFRI, SUI), Tolinase (AUS, BEL, ESP, HOL, SUI, SWE, USA).

13. *Muscle relaxants*

Aneural (FRG), Carisoma (GBR), Dantamacrin (FRG), Dantrium (AUS, BEL, CAN, FRA, GBR, HOL, NZL, S.AFRI, USA), Distalene (ARG), Equanil (AUS, CAN, DEN, FRA, GBR, S.AFRI, USA), Flexeril (CAN, USA), Lyseen (ARG, BEL, FRG), Maolate (USA), Methocabal (JPN), Mydocalm (DEN, FRA, HOL, HUN, SUI), Norflex (AUS, BEL, CAN, DEN, FRG, GBR, S.AFRI, SUI, SWE, USA), Rinlaxer (JPN), Robaxin (ARG, AUS, CAN, DEN, GBR, HOL, NOR, S.AFRI, SWE, SUI, USA), Sinaxar (AUS, BEL, DEN, S.AFRI), Soma (CAN, ITA, USA).

14. *Ointments/creams/lotions*

Baciguent (CAN, USA), Bacitracin (—), Caladryl (GBR), Debrisan (AUS, DEN, GBR, HOL, NOR, NZL, S.AFRI, SWE, USA), Iduviran (FRA, SUI), Myciguent (AUS, CAN, S.AFRI, USA), Neosporin (GBR), Retin-A (AUX, GBR, ITA, NZL, S.AFRI, SUI, USA), Soframycin (AUS, CAN, DEN, GBR, HOL, S.AFRI, SUI), Stoxil (AUS, CAN, S.AFRI, USA), Vioform (AUS, CAN, FRG, GBR, S.AFRI, SUI, USA), Zostrum (EIRE, FRG).

15. *Ophthalmic and otic preparations*

Albucid (ARG, AUS, GBR, S.AFRI), Auralgen (—), Auraltone (GBR), Collyrium (GBR), Disine (AUS, GBR, ITA, SUI, USA), Iduviran (FRA, SUI), Maxitrol (GBR), Myciquent (AUS, CAN, S.AFRI, USA), Opticrom (AUS, CAN, FRG, GBR, NZL, SUI), Ototrips (GBR), Otrivine-Antistin (GBR), Phenazone (ARG, AUS, BEL, BRA, HUN, JAP, MEX, POL, RUS, TCH, USA), Polyfax (GBR), Prontamid (ITA),

Sodium Sulamyd (CAN, USA), Vasosulf (S.AFRI), Xerumenex (GBR).

117

Chapter 6
Uses and abuses
of drugs in sport:
the athlete's view

16. Penicillins and other antibiotics

Achromycin (AUS, CAN, DEN, FRG, GBR, HOL, NOR, S.AFRI, SUI, SWE, USA), Amikin (AUS, CAN, EIRE, S.AFRI, SUI, USA), Amoxidal (ARG), Amoxypen (FRG), Bacitracin (—), Bactramin (JPN), Bactrim (ARG, AUS, BEL, CAN, DEN, FRA, FRG, GBR, ITA, NOR, S.AFRI, SUI, SWE, USA), Biklin (ARG, DEN, FRG, JPN, SWE), Brulamycin (HUN), Ceclor (CAN, USA), Cefro (JPN), Clamoxyl (BEL, ESP, FRA, FRG, HOL, JPN, SUI), Cloxapen (CAN, ITA, USA), Erythrocyn (AUS, CAN, FRG, S.AFRI, USA), Espectrin (BRA, HKG, MAL), Floxapen (AUS, BEL, GBR, HOL, ITA, NZL, S.AFRI, SUI), Fosfocin (FRA, ITA), Gantrisen (AUS, BEL, CAN, DEN, FRG, GBR, HOL, S.AFRI, SWE, USA), Garamycin (AUS, CAN, DEN, GBR, HOL, NOR, S.AFRI, SUI, USA), Keflex (AUS, CAN, DEN, GBR, JPN, NOR, S.AFRI, SUI, USA), Kefzol (AUS, BEL, CAN, DEN, FRA, GBR, HOL, S.AFRI, SUI, USA), Lemandine (ESP), Mandelamine (AUS, BEL, FRG, S.AFRI, SUI, USA), Mandokef (DEN, ESP, FRG, S.AFRI), Mandol (AUS, CAN, HOL, NZL, USA), Minocin (BEL, CAN, ESP, HOL, ITA, SUI, USA), Minomycin (AUS, JAP, S.AFRI), Nebcin(e) (AUS, CAN, S.AFRI, USA), Orbenin (AUS, BEL, CAN, ESP, GBR, HOL, ITA, S.AFRI, SUI), Oroxin (JPN), Panoral (FRG), Penbritin (ARG, AUS, BEL, CAN, HOL, S.AFRI, SUI, USA), Pentrex (S.AFRI), Purmycin (S.AFRI), Pyassan (HUN), Rondamycin (AUS, GBR, SUI, SWE, USA), Roscillin (IND), Semicillin (HUN), Taimoxin (JPN), Tobra (ARG), Totacillin (JPN), Ultramycin (CAN), Velocef (ARG, ESP, ITA), Veramina (ARG), Vibramycin (AUS, CAN, DEN, FRG, GBR, JPN, NOR, S.AFRI, SUI, USA).

17. Phenytoin and some other anticonvulsants

Celontin (AUS, BEL, CAN, ITA, S.AFRI, USA), Depakene (JPN, USA), Depakine (ITA), Dilantin (AUS, CAN, USA), Dilon (ARG), Epamin (ARG), Epanutin (BEL, ESP, FRG, GBR, HOL, NOR, S.AFRI, SUI, SWE), Gardenal (BEL, CAN, ESP, FRA, ITA, S.AFRI), Hermolepsin (SWE), Hydantol (JPN), Iktorivil (SWE), Majsolin (YUG), Mysoline (AUS, BEL, CAN, DEN, FRA, ITA, NOR, S.AFRI, SUI, USA), Neuracen (FRG), Nidrane (ARG, AUS, GBR), Ospolot (AUS, DEN, ESP, FRG, GBR, HOL, ITA, S.AFRI), Paradoine (AUS, BEL, CAN, FRA, USA), Peganone (AUS, DEN, NOR, SUI, SWE, USA), Phenobarbital (—), Prosoline (ISR), Rivotril (ARG, AUS, BEL, CAN, DEN, FRA, FRG, GBR, HOL, ITA, NOR, S.AFRI, USA), Tegretol (ARG, AUS, BEL, CAN, DEN, FRA, GBR, HOL, ITA, NOR, S.AFRI, SUI, USA), Timonil (FRG), Tridione (AUS, BEL, DEN,

118

Chapter 6
Uses and abuses
of drugs in sport:
the athlete's view

FRG, GBR, S.AFRI, USA), Zarontin (ARG, AUS, BEL, CAN, ESP, FRA, GBR, ITA, S.AFRI, USA).

18. *Promethazine and other antihistamines*

Actidil (AUS, CAN, DEN, ITA, S.AFRI), Actidilon (ARG, FRA), Allergex (S.AFRI), Alusas (JPN), Anthisan (AUS, DEN, GBR, NOR, S.AFRI), Antistin(e) (CAN, ESP, FRA, FRG, SUI), Astemizole (CAN), Atalis-D (JPN), Atarax (ARG, AUS, CAN, FRG, USA), Atosil (FRG), Avomine (AUS, S.AFRI), Azaron (HOL), Banistyl (AUS, S.AFRI), Bonpac (JPN), C-Meton-S (JPN), Chlorpheniramine (—), Chlor-Tripolon (CAN, USA), Clistin (ARG, AUS, ITA, USA), Dimetane (AUS, CAN, ESP, S.AFRI), Di-Paralene (AUS, BEL, FRA, ITA), Ebalin (FRG), Fabhistin (AUS, GBR, S.AFRI), Hismanal (CAN), Histalert (AUS, S.AFRI), Histantil (CAN), Histex (AUS), Histryl (AUS, BEL, S.AFRI), Homadamon (JPN), Idulamine (ARG), Ifrasarl (JPN), Incidal (HOL, ITA), Lecasol (JPN), Lenazine (S.AFRI), Migristene (ARG, BEL, FRA, FRG, JPN), Nuran (FRG), Omeril (FRG), Optimine (CAN, HOL, S.AFRI, USA), Periactin (ARG, BEL, CAN, S.AFRI), Peritol (HUN), Phenergan (AUS, BEL, CAN, FRA, S.AFRI, SUI), Polaronil (FRG), Prof-N-4 (ARG), Promaquid (CAN), Pyribenzamine (CAN), Pyrimetane (ARG), Reconin (JPN), Sacronal (JPN), Seldane (CAN), Tavegyl (ARG, BEL, HUN, S.AFRI, SUI), Tavist (CAN), Teldane (FRA), Trihistan (DEN, NOR, SUI), Triluden (CAN), Trimeton (ITA), Venen (JPN).

Beware

Use only plain preparations. Combinations often contain banned drugs like codeine, ephedrine, phenylpropanolamine, etc.

19. *Purgatives (laxatives or cathartics)*

Adjust (JPN), Alaxa (ITA), Anan (JPN), Bancon (ITA), Bekunis (FRG, JPN), Co-lace (CAN, USA), Dialose (USA), Dorbanex (GBR, SWE), Dulcolax (BEL, CAN, DEN, FRA, FRG, GBR, HOL, ITA, NOR, S.AFRI, SUI, SWE, USA), Eulaxan (FRG), Lunelax (SWE), Metamucil (CAN, GBR, HOL, USA), Milk of magnesia (—), Normalax (SWE), Senokot (AUS, BEL, CAN, ESP, FRA, GBR, USA).

20. *Vaginal preparations*

Betadine (AUS, CAN, ESP, FRA, GBR, HOL, S.AFRI, SUI, USA), Candeptin (CAN, S.AFRI, SWE), Deflamon (ITA), Empecid (ARG, JPN), Entizol (POL), Eparol (GBR), Flagyl (ARG, AUS, BEL, CAN, DEN, ESP, FRA, FRG, GBR, ITA, NOR, NZL, S.AFRI, SUI, SWE, USA), Floraquin (ARG, AUS, BEL), Gyno-Pevaryl (BEL, FRA, FRG,

119

Chapter 6
Uses and abuses
of drugs in sport:
the athlete's view

GBR, HOL, NOR, NZL, S.AFRI, SUI), Klion (HUN), Nida (JPN), Monistat (CAN, GBR, SUI, USA), Mycostatin (ARG, AUS, CAN, DEN, ESP, FRA, ITA, NOR, S.AFRI, SUI, USA), Pimafucin (AUS, BEL, DEN, FRG, GBR, HOL, ITA, NOR, S.AFRI, SUI), Vanobid (USA).

21. Vitamins and mineral preparations

Beware

All vitamins and minerals are permitted. Some so-called 'vitamins' preparations may contain banned drugs, such as psychomotor stimulants and anabolic steroids.

Part II: Generic names of preparations listed in Part I

1. Antacids and some other gastrointestinal agents like anti-diarrhoeals

Alginic acid
Aluminium glycinate
Aluminium hydroxide (dried)
Aluminium hodroxide−magnesium carbonate co-dried gel
Bismuth subsalicylate and methyl salicylate
Calcium carbonate
Dimethicone (activated)
Diphenoxylate hydrochloride
Hydrotalcite (aluminium magnesium hydroxide carbonate hydrate)
Hyoscyamine sulphate
Kaolin (hydrated aluminium silicate)
Loperamide hydrochloride
Magaldrate (hydrated magnesium aluminate)
Magnesium carbonate (light)
Mebeverine
Mepenzolate bromide
Neomycin sulphate
Proglumide
Sucralfate

2. Anti-asthmatic agents and anti-allergenic agents

Aminophylline
Beclomethasone Diproprionate*
Bitolterol*
Choline theophyllinate
Ipratropium bromide
Orciprenaline*

120

Chapter 6
Uses and abuses
of drugs in sport:
the athlete's view

Rimiterol*
Salbutamol*
Sodium Chromoglycate
Terbutaline*
Theophylline
*Note: the use of these substances is allowed by inhalation only.

3. Anti-nauseants and anti-emetic agents

Dimenhydrinate
Diphenidol
Hyoscine
Invert sugar
Meclozine

Metoclopramide
Prochlorperazine
Scopolamine
Triethylperazine
Trimethobenzamide

4. Anti-ulcer drugs

Burimamide
Carbenoxolane
Cimetidine

Metiamide
Metoclopramide
Ranitidine

5. Aspirin and similar analgesic (non-narcotic) and anti-inflammatory non-steroidal agents

Acetylcresotinic acid
Acetylsalicylic acid (aspirin)
Alclofenac
Aloxiprin
Aluminium aspirin
Azapropazone
Benorylate
Benzydamine
Bucolome
Bufexamac
Calcium
Carbaspirin
Diclofenac
Difenamizole
Diflunisal
Fenbufen

Fendosal
Floctafenine
Flufenamic acid
Glafenine
Ibuprofen
Indomethacin
Indoprofen
Ketoprofen
Mefenamic acid
Naproxen
Oxyphenbutazone
Paracetamol (acetaminophen)
Piroxicam
Sodium salicylate
Sulindac
Tolmetin

6. Contraceptives

Ethynodiol diacetate and ethinyloestradiol
Ethynodiol diacetate and mestranol
Lenonorgestrel and ethinyloestradiol
Lynoestrenol and ethinyloestradiol

Lynoestrenol and Mestranol
Norethisterone and ethinyloestradiol
Norethisterone and Mestranol

121

Chapter 6
Uses and abuses
of drugs in sport:
the athlete's view

7. Decongestants and nasal preparations

Beclomethasone
  dipropionate
Framycetin
Naphazoline

Oxymetazoline
Tetrahydrozoline
Xylometazoline

8. Expectorants and cough suppressants

Syrups

Bromhexine
Dextromethorphan
Guaiphenesin
Pholcodine

Suppositories

Cineol
Gaiacol
Morclofone

Tablets

Benzonatate
Bibenzonium
Bromhexine
Butamyrate citrate
Cloperastine
Dimemorfan
Zipeprol

9. Griseofulvin and other antifungal agents

Amphotericin
Chlormidazole
Clotrimazole
Flucytosine
Griseofulvin

Miconazole
Natamycin
Nystatin
Tinidazole
Tolnaftate

10. Haemorrhoidal preparations

Aluminium acetate
Benzocaine
Benzyl benzoate
Bismuth (oxide, subgallate)
Boric acid
Butyl aminobenzoate
Cinchocaine
Esculoside
Framycetin
Hexachlorophane

Hydrocortisone
Lignocaine
Neomycin
Peru Balsam
Polymyxin B sulphate
Pramoxine
Resorcine
Resorcinol
Zinc oxide

122

Chapter 6
Uses and abuses
of drugs in sport:
the athlete's view

11. Hypnotics, sedatives and tranquillisers

Acetylcarbromal
Amylobarbitone
Bromazepam
Butobarbitone
Carbromal
Chloral hydrate
Chlorpromazine hydrochloride
Chlordiazepoxide
Clorazepate dipotassium
Diazepam
Dichloralphenazone
Ethinamate
Flurazepam
Glutethimide
Haloperidol
Heptabarbitone
Hexobarbitone
Hexobarbitone and
    cyclobarbitone
Lorazepam
Meprobamate
Methaqualone
Methylphenobarbitone
Methyprylen
Nitrazepam
Oxazepam
Pentobarbitone
Phenobarbitone
Quinalbarbitone
Temazepam
Triazolam
Trifluoperazine

12. Insulin and other antidiabetic agents

Acetohexamide
Buformin
Carbutamide
Chlorpropamide
Glibenclamide
Glibornuride
Gliclazide
Glybuzole
Insulin
Metformin
Phenformin
Tolazamide
Tolbutamide

13. Muscle relaxants

Carisoprodol
Chlorphenesin
Cyclobenzaprine
Dantrolene
Meprobamate
Methocarbamol
Orphenadrine
Prydenol
Styramate
Tolperisone

14. Ointment, creams, lotions

Bacitracin
Calamine
Clioquinol
Dextranomer
Dimethicone
Diphenhydramine
Framycetin
Idoxuridine
Neomycin
Tretinoin

123

*Chapter 6
Uses and abuses
of drugs in sport:
the athlete's view*

15. Ophthalmic and otic preparations

Acetic acid
Antazoline
Antipyrine
Bacitracin
Benzocaine
Borate solution (neutral)
Chlorbutol
Dexamethasone
Idoxuridine
Naphazoline
Neomycin
Oxyquinoline

Phenazone
Pilocarpine
Polymyxin B sulphate
Sodium cromoglycate
Sulphacetamide sodium
Tetrahydrozoline
Triethanolamine polypeptide
    oleate condensate
Trypsin
Xylometazoline
Zine sulphate

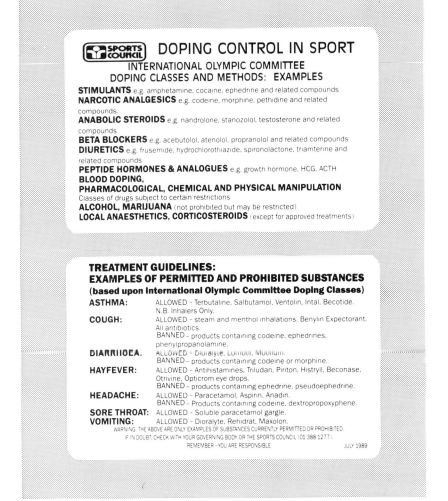

SPORTS COUNCIL DOPING CONTROL IN SPORT
INTERNATIONAL OLYMPIC COMMITTEE
DOPING CLASSES AND METHODS: EXAMPLES

STIMULANTS e.g. amphetamine, cocaine, ephedrine and related compounds
NARCOTIC ANALGESICS e.g. codeine, morphine, pethidine and related compounds.
ANABOLIC STEROIDS e.g. nandrolone, stanozolol, testosterone and related compounds
BETA BLOCKERS e.g. acebutolol, atenolol, propranolol and related compounds
DIURETICS e.g. frusemide, hydrochlorothiazide, spironolactone, triamterine and related compounds
PEPTIDE HORMONES & ANALOGUES e.g. growth hormone, HCG, ACTH
BLOOD DOPING,
PHARMACOLOGICAL, CHEMICAL AND PHYSICAL MANIPULATION
Classes of drugs subject to certain restrictions
ALCOHOL, MARIJUANA (not prohibited but may be restricted)
LOCAL ANAESTHETICS, CORTICOSTEROIDS (except for approved treatments)

TREATMENT GUIDELINES:
EXAMPLES OF PERMITTED AND PROHIBITED SUBSTANCES
(based upon International Olympic Committee Doping Classes)

ASTHMA: ALLOWED - Terbutaline, Salbutamol, Ventolin, Intal, Becotide. N.B. Inhalers Only.
COUGH: ALLOWED - steam and menthol inhalations. Benylin Expectorant. All antibiotics.
BANNED - products containing codeine, ephedrines, phenylpropanolamine.
DIARRHOEA: ALLOWED - Dioralyte, Lomotil, Motilium.
BANNED - products containing codeine or morphine.
HAYFEVER: ALLOWED - Antihistamines, Triludan, Piriton, Histryll, Beconase, Otrivine, Opticrom eye drops.
BANNED - products containing ephedrine, pseudoephedrine.
HEADACHE: ALLOWED - Paracetamol, Aspirin, Anadin.
BANNED - Products containing codeine, dextropropoxyphene.
SORE THROAT: ALLOWED - Soluble paracetamol gargle.
VOMITING: ALLOWED - Dioralyte, Rehidrat, Maxolon.
WARNING: THE ABOVE ARE ONLY EXAMPLES OF SUBSTANCES CURRENTLY PERMITTED OR PROHIBITED.
IF IN DOUBT, CHECK WITH YOUR GOVERNING BODY OR THE SPORTS COUNCIL (01 388 1277).
REMEMBER -YOU ARE RESPONSIBLE   JULY 1989

Card issued to sports men and women summarizing substances banned by the IOC.
(From the Sports Council.)

124

Chapter 6
Uses and abuses
of drugs in sport:
the athlete's view

16. Penicillins and other antibiotics

Amikacin
Amoxycillin
Ampicillin
Bacitracin
Cefaclor
Cephalexin
Cephamandalate
Cephazoline
Cephradine
Cloxacillin
Co-Trimoxazole
Doxycycline

Erythromycin
Flucloxacillin
Fosfomycin
Gentamicin
Hexamine
Methacycline
Minocycline
Penicillin
Sulphafurazole
Tetracycline
Tobramycin

17. Phenytoin and some other anticonvulsants

Beclamide
Carbamazepine
Clonazepam
Ethosuximide
Ethotoin
Methsuximide
Paramethadione

Phenobarbitone
Phenytoin
Primidone
Sulthiame
Trixidone
Valproic acid

18. Promethazine and other antihistamines

Antazoline
Astemizole
Azatadine
Brompheniramine
Carbinoxamine
Chlorcyclizine
Chlorpheniramine
Clemastine
Cyproheptadine
Dexchlorpheniramine

Dimethothiazine
Diphenylpyraline
Homochlorcyclizine
Hydroxyzine
Mebhydrolin
Mepyramine
Promethazine
Terfenadine
Tripelennamine
Triprolidine

19. Purgatives (laxatives or cathartics)

Bisacodyl
Danthron
Docusate
Ispaghula Husk

Magnesium hydroxide
Phenolphtalol
Tinnevelly Senna Fruit

125
Chapter 6
Uses and abuses
of drugs in sport:
the athlete's view

20. Vaginal preparations

Benzoyl metronidazole
Candicidin
Clotrimazole
Di-iodohydroxyquinoline
Econazole

Metronidazole
Miconazole
Natamycin
Nystalin

21. Vitamins and mineral preparations

Vitamins A, B, C, D, E, and others.

References

Anstiss T. J. (1989) Returning after injury — who makes the decision? *Coaching Focus* **11**, 7–8.
Buick E. J., Gledhill N., Froese A. B., Spriet L. & Meyers E. C. (1976) Effect of induced erythrocythaemia on aerobic work capacity. *Journal of Applied Physiology* **40**, 379–83.
Bullock W., White A. & Worthington J. (1968) The effects of anabolic steroids on amino acid incorporation by skeletal muscle ribosomes. *Biochemistry Journal* **108**, 417–25.
Donohue T. & Johnson N. (1986) *Foul Play — Drug Abuse in Sport*. Basil Blackwell, Oxford.
Gledhill N. (1982) Blood doping and related issues: a brief review. *Medicine, Science Sport and Exercise* **14**(3), 183–9.
Goodman A. G. & Gilman, A. *The Pharmacological Basis of Therapeutics*, 6th edn. Ballière Tindall, London.
Haupt H. & Rovere G. (1984) Anabolic steroids: a review of the literature. *American Journal of Sports Medicine* **12**(6), 469–84.
Heere L. P. (1988) Piroxicam in acute musculoskeletal disorders and sports injuries. *American Journal of Sports Medicine* **84**, 50–55.
Kruse P. (1986) Beta-blockade used in precision sports: effects on pistol shooting performance. *Journal of Applied Physiology* **61**(2), 417–20.
Kibble M. & Ross M. (1987) Drug review. *Clinical Pharmacy* **6**, 687.
MacIntyre J. (1987) Growth hormone and athletes. *Sports Medicine* **4**, 129–42.
Mandell A. J. (1976) The *Nightmare Season*. New York: Random House.
Mandell A. J. (1979) The Sunday syndrome: a unique pattern of amphetamine abuse indigenous to American professional football. *Clinical Toxicology* **15**(2), 225–32.
Medical news and perspectives (1987) *Journal of the American Medical Association* **257**(22), 3021–5.
Murray T. (1983) The coercive power of drugs in sport. *The Hastings Center Report*. New York, pp. 24–30.
Neff C. (1983) Caracas: A scandal and a warning. *Sports Illustrated* **59**, 18–19.
Pope G. & Katz D. (1988) Affective and psychotic symptoms in anabolic steroid users. *American Journal of Psychiatry* **145**(4), 487–90.
Prokop L. (1970) The struggle against doping and its history. *Journal of Sports Medicine and Physical Fitness* **10**(1), 45–8.
Roy S. & Irvin R. (1983) *Sports Medicine, Prevention, Evaluation, Management and Rehabilitation*. New Jersey: Prentice Hall.
Silverman F. (1984) Guaranteed aggression: The secret use of testosterone by Nazi troops. *Journal of the American Medical Association*, May, 129–31.
Silvester J. (1973) Anabolic steroids and the Munich Olympics. *Scholastic Coach* **43**, 90–2.
Taylor W. (1987) Synthetic anabolic–androgenic steroids: a plea for controlled substance status. *Physician and Sports Medicine* **15**(5), 140–50.
Thomson J. M., Stone J. A., Ginsburg A. D. & Hamilton P. (1983) The effects of blood reinfusion during prolonged, heavy exercise. *Canadian Journal of Applied Sports Science* **8**(2), 72–8.
Todd T. (1983) The steroid predicament. *Sports Illustrated* **59**, 63–77.
Todd T. (1987) Anabolic steroids: the gremlins of sport. *Journal of Sport History* **14**(1), 87–107.

7 The case against anabolic steroids

I. S. BENJAMIN

'He thought he saw a kangaroo that worked a coffee mill
He looked again and found it was a vegetable pill
Were I to swallow this he said I should be very ill'
From *Silvie and Bruno* by Lewis Caroll

The use of anabolic steroids to improve performance in sport has been known for 30 years, but has gained both momentum and notoriety during the last decade. General aspects of the use and abuse of drugs in sport have been discussed in a previous chapter (Chapter 6). This chapter will concentrate in detail on the history of developments in the use of anabolic and androgenic steroids, their desirable and undesirable effects, and the case against their use.

Biochemistry and physiology

Testosterone is the basic steroid molecule on which all of these compounds are based. It is secreted by interstitial cells of the testis in man, and is responsible for development of the male secondary sexual characteristics at puberty. Testosterone is metabolised in the liver to the less potent androsterone and dihydroepiandrosterone, which are conjugated and excreted in the urine. Testosterone was first successfully synthesised in 1935. In its native form it is ineffective when administered by mouth, largely because of hepatic metabolism. Numerous synthetic substances such as methyltestosterone, however, are effective as oral preparations.

The effects of these hormones are both androgenic and anabolic. Their androgenic effects in males include trophic actions on the activity of spermatozoa, as well as development of the accessory sexual organs. Exogenous androgens will obviate the deficiencies of pre-pubertal testicular underdevelopment, and will reverse the effects of post-pubertal castration. Endogenous testosterone is also largely responsible for the male emotional make-up.

The second group of activities is anabolic, promoting nitrogen retention and increased synthesis and deposition of protein in numerous tissues, especially in skeletal muscle. Since it is the anabolic effects which are sought by athletes, it is in the manifestation of undesirable androgenic effects that the weakness of these substances lies. Attempts have been made to produce related compounds in which anabolic activity is enhanced at the expense of androgenic

126

activity, but these have only been partially successful. Modification of the side-chains of the steroid molecule produces compounds
such as norethandrolone and methandrostenolone (Dianabol), compounds which possess both enhanced anabolic potency and oral
availability.

History of steroid use

In 1889 the French physiologist Brown-Séquard, believing old age
and its associated dwindling of sexual powers to be reversible by
agents contained in the testis, injected himself with crushed guinea-
pig testes. He reported to the Société Biologie in Paris that these
injections had proved effective, but his personal observations were
greeted with some hostility and scepticism. However, such is the
susceptibility of the public to this powerful suggestion that his
report laid open the way to Voronoff's celebrated xenotransplanta-
tion of monkey testis slices, which swept America and Europe
during the 1920s (Hamilton 1986).

Following the synthesis of testosterone in 1935 the substance
was said to have been used to enhance the aggressiveness of German
soldiers during World War II. If this account is not simply apocry-
phal, it was an interesting twist of fate which led to the use of these
steroids in the treatment of survivors of concentration camps at the
end of that war.

Probably the first use of anabolic steroids by atheletes was in the
1950s, when weight-lifters sought to increase strength and bulk by
the use of injectable synthetic testosterone. By the 1956 Olympics
in Melbourne, many athletes were using methandrostenolone (Dianabol), an oral steroid with a higher anabolic : androgenic ratio (Bierly
1987). At this time steroids had not yet been included on the list
of banned substances by the International Olympic Committee, a
move which did not take place until the 1976 Games in Montreal,
at which event six athletes were positive when tested for steroids.
Since that time the use of steroid has been detected in increasing
numbers of athletes, with disqualification of 15 athletes, and withdrawals by several more, from the Pan-American Games in Caracas,
Venezuela, in 1983. In the 1984 Olympics in Los Angeles silver
medals were lost in the 10 000 m and wrestling events for the same
reason.

Spread from these high echelons of sporting achievement to the
American College Football scene was recognised in 1987. In this
year the National Collegiate Athletic Association tested 720 football players at the end of the season, and suspended twenty-one who
tested positive. In 1988 the former British sprinter David Jenkins
was found guilty on charges of steroid trafficking in the USA, and
the scale of the problem became much more apparent. In the same
year at the Seoul Olympics in Korea the battle between the athletes

and the biochemists was brought to the newspaper headlines of the world by the stripping of Ben Johnson's gold medal in the 100 m event. By this stage there could be nobody with an interest in sport, medicine, law or ethics who was unaware of the phenomenon.

When it comes to estimating the scale of the problem, the matter becomes more complex. Informal surveys of athletes, particularly those in sports requiring either great bulk and strength or explosive power, have suggested that as many as 90% of those in serious training have used steroids at one time or another. Formal statistics are much less easy to achieve. A survey of amateur body-builders in a Scottish gymnasium was performed by McKillop (1987). Eight out of forty-one (19.5%) admitted to the use of drugs to enhance their performance, and most of these were anabolic steroids. All the users had taken combinations of drugs, and in no case had there been any medical supervision.

The same problem of gathering reliable statistics for what is a widely practised but illegal activity has also meant that any form of controlled trial for the use of steroids has been impossible. While some team physicians in the USA have said that they think steroid use is declining, one experienced observer stated that 'every professional football player I know takes them, with some position-related exceptions' (Wright 1987).

Do anabolic steroids work?

The evidence that anabolic steroids can in fact increase muscle mass and power is inconclusive. Lamb (1984) reviewed nineteen studies in which some form of control was available. Twelve of these studies showed that weight gains averaging 2.2 kg over a period of three to 12 weeks were attained by athletes taking methandro-stenolone. While some of this gain may be due to increased fluid retention, there probably was also a substantial increase in lean body mass. In addition, approximately half of these controlled investigations showed that there was a progressive improvement in muscular strength when steroids were taken along with highly intensive weight-training. Athletes taking steroids typically achieved gains over those taking placebo which averaged 8 kg for single repetition maximum lifts in the bench-press and 11 kg in the squat.

An important physiological observation must be made in relation to these studies. Those athletes who gain a major beneficial effect from the use of anabolic steroids are invariably those already engaged in the most rigorous levels of physical training. The reason for this is that the anabolic effects of exogenous steroids are intrinsically very short-lived. Thus, little or no benefit may be gained by subjects in a neutral state of metabolism. However, intensively training athletes induce in themselves a persistent catabolic state, mediated by high levels of glucocorticoids resulting from increased

ACTH stimulation. A weight-lifter in intensive training may have difficulty in consuming enough protein (2–2.2 g/kg per day) to maintain positive nitrogen balance, and may thus be in a chronically catabolic state. It is the anticatabolic effect of steroids which may therefore allow these athletes to train at such intensive levels and still maintain the required protein anabolism (Haupt & Rovere 1984). Sadly, this message may not always reach susceptible young persons who may be tempted to try to achieve rapid result by pharmacology rather than by hard training.

Finally, it must be admitted that not all of the beneficial effects of anabolic steroids in training athletes are critically dependent on physiological changes. One of the principal effects reported by those using these drugs is increased physical tolerance to training and more rapid recovery from heavy training sessions. This may indeed be a physical effect, but may also have a strong psychological component. Moreover, the increased aggressiveness which is undoubtedly one of the effects of steroids may itself make a major contribution to the athlete's performance. The search for evidence from controlled trials for or against the physical effects of steroids is doomed to failure. Most clinical trials in medicine are aimed at demonstrating differences between groups of at least 10%. By contrast, an improvement in performance of only 1–2% may represent the margin between victory and defeat in international athletic events. It has been pointed out in a recent leading article that 'no negative trial is likely to be as convincing to athletes as Ben Johnson's performance in the Olympic 100 metre final' (BMJ 1988).

Undesirable effects of steroids

Cardiovascular system

Anabolic steroids cause fluid retention, which may in part account for the early weight gain during their use. Significant increases in blood pressure occur along with left ventricular hypertrophy. Changes in lipoproteins have been observed during several studies. In training athletes the ratio of low density to high density lipoproteins is reduced, and this is said to be one of the factors which lowers the risk of ischaemic heart disease in athletes. However, this relationship may be reversed by the use of anabolic steroids, by a ratio of almost four to one (Lenders *et al.* 1988). There has been one report of acute myocardial infarction in a 22-year-old world class weight-lifter who used anabolic steroids (McNutt *et al.* 1988).

Coagulation

Many steroids increase levels of clotting factors, particularly Factors V, X and prothrombin. In addition the drugs may induce polycythaemia and also have generalised oestrogenic effects. Increased coagulability increases the risk of arterial occlusion and there has been one case report of a stroke occurring in a 34-year-old body-builder (Frankle *et al.* 1988).

Male reproductive system

Testosterone and its analogues cause suppression of follicular-stimulating hormone and luteinising hormone. This will result in testicular atrophy, oligospermia and azoospermia. Gynaecomastia is a frequent finding, and one paper reported thirty-eight surgical procedures for this condition in body-builders (Aiache 1989). In addition, adenocarcinoma of the prostate has been reported in a 40-year-old bodybuilder (Roberts & Essenhigh 1986).

Female reproductive system

Uterine atrophy and menstrual irregularity are common, making pregnancy unlikely. However, if steroids are taken during pregnancy, pseudohermaphroditism or fetal death are both hazards. Amongst the secondary sexual changes in women, acne, deepening of the voice, facial hair and baldness, shrinkage of the breast and clitoral hypertrophy contribute to the rather unattractive features. Major stimulation of the sebaceous glands occurs in either sex (Kiraly *et al.* 1987).

Effects in children

Before closure of the epiphyseal plates, steroids will cause premature fusion with permanent stunting of growth. In adolescence, extreme virilisation may occur, along with gynaecomastia. Decreased spermatogenesis and sterility occur, though these changes may be reversible. These effects are particularly worrying as the pressure to use anabolic steroids penetrates to younger age groups, with particular influences having been noted in high school children in the USA (*Baltimore Evening Sun*, 8 June 1987). A survey carried out amongst high school athletes in the USA showed only minimal use of steroids (1% of 295 students) and amphetamines (2%). However, 32% of males and 13% of females believed that steroids were effective, and 14% of males (but no females) said they would consider using these agents. There seemed to be little understanding in this group of the real hazards of steroids (Krowchuk *et al.* 1989).

Psychological effects

These include wild swings in mood and unpredictable aggressive behaviour. There have been reports of criminal activity resulting from these psychological disturbances. Changes in libido are also common, and may contribute to the impotence reported by some male athletes using steroids.

Effects on the liver

Abnormal results of liver function tests are common, with increased transaminases, alkaline phosphatase, lactate dehydrogenase and bilirubin during administration. In severe cases a cholestatic hepatitis may occur. These changes are generally reversible on withdrawing the steroids, and have to be distinguished from the elevation of transaminases which may occur with intense weight-lifting alone.

Most of the hepatic side-effects of anabolic steroids have been reported in patients receiving these preparations for therapeutic purposes. Treatment with androgenic and anabolic steroids has proved effective in the management of Fanconi's anaemia, a rare genetic disorder resulting in pancytopaenia along with a number of growth disorders. The natural history of the disease is death from anaemia or sepsis within one or two years. Liver disease associated with such treatment was first reported in 1965 by Recant and Lacey and was followed in 1971 by a report from Bernstein *et al.* of both hepatoma and peliosis hepatis (a rare condition characterised by blood-filled cystic spaces within the liver) in a Fanconi patient under treatment. In a review article in 1983 Westaby *et al.* reported 33 cases of androgen-associated hepatic tumours, 14 being treated for Fanconi's anaemia and nineteen for other conditions. They added three cases of their own, all receiving therapeutic androgens. The range of liver lesions found in patients treated with anabolic steroids include generalised hyperplasia, hyperplastic nodules, liver cell adenoma, and hepatocellular carcinoma (Sweeney & Evans 1976). This suggests there may be a common mechanism for these abnormalities mediated by a stimulus to hepatocyte hyperplasia, although cholangiocarcinoma has also been reported with anabolic steroid therapy (Stromeyer *et al.* 1979).

All of these reports have been in patients receiving anabolic steroids for therapy. However, in 1984 Overly *et al.* reported the case of a 26-year-old body-builder who had taken a number of androgenic and anabolic steroids over a period of four years. He presented with weight loss and malaise, and was found to have a massive hepatic tumour with both cholangiocellular and hepatocellular elements, and with both intra-abdominal and pulmonary metastases. This important report was the first case of fatal hepatocellular disease in an athlete associated with androgenic steroid abuse. We have seen a similar case at Hammersmith Hospital.

Case report

David Singh was a 27-year-old body-builder who had taken inter-mittent courses of anabolic steroids (the preparations used are not known) over several years. He presented to a District Hospital with sudden onset of severe abdominal and left shoulder pain, which initially improved but progressed to collapse and admission to hospital in a shocked state. Laparotomy was performed and 2 litres of blood were found in the peritoneal cavity from spontaneous rupture of the right liver. The abdomen was packed and the patient transferred to Hammersmith Hospital, where on arrival there were signs of continued bleeding. Visceral angiography showed a diffusely abnormal circulation in the right liver with a tumour blush, and a working diagnosis of spontaneous rupture of a hepatic adenoma was made. Because there were signs of continued bleeding urgent laparotomy was undertaken, and a rupture in the dome of the right liver was found. There were several other nodules palpable in the liver, and the whole texture of the organ was grossly abnormal, friable and soft. Mobilization of the right liver was performed for a hepatectomy, but it was found that the ruptured main tumour mass involved the inferior vena cava, and despite all operative efforts uncontrollable haemorrhage ended in death on the operating table.

At autopsy, examination of the resected right liver and the residual left liver revealed four nodules ranging from 5 to 40 mm in diameter, the largest of these showing signs of extensive haemorrhage. The whole liver was the site of diffuse hepatocyte hyperplasia and peliosis hepatis. Histological examination showed that the nodules were hepatocellular adenomas but the largest of these showed histological evidence of malignant transformation (Creagh *et al.* 1988).

A coroner's inquest returned a verdict which drew a cause and effect association between the steroids and the ruptured liver which led to this young man's death (Daily Telegraph, 1 July 1987), and the coroner described the case as 'almost unique'.

Detection of drugs

Detection of drugs used to enhance sporting performance has become a new major industry. Workers at the Olympic Analytical Laboratory in Los Angeles reported in 1987 that they had conducted 8000 tests for androgenic anabolic steroids over a three year period, and found several hundred positive cases (Hatton & Catlin 1987). The same authors noted that during the 1984 Los Angeles Olympic Games almost 10 000 analyses were performed during a 15-day period, covering more than 200 different drugs and metabolites, with only a 2% positivity rate (Catlin *et al.* 1987). Rosenbloom and Sutton (1985) have pointed out that the drug testing facilities used for the 1984 Olympics cost more to operate than the total athletics budget of many countries.

The scope and nature of drug testing in athletes has received increasing attention during the last decade, and the publicity surrounding the Seoul Olympics in 1988 has sharpened both public and medical attention on this topic (Cowart 1989). The need to set detection levels at such a point that there are no false positives may result in many athletes who are using drugs being able to beat the testers readily. One example is the method used for detection of testosterone abuse. This is detected by measurement of the ratio of testosterone : epitestosterone in the urine. In normal men this is between 1:1 and 1:2.5, and the level set by the International Olympic Committee is 1:6. However, it is very easy to devise a dosage of testosterone such that a ratio of 1:6 is never exceeded, as proved in a trial of administration to military volunteers for six weeks (Cowart 1989). The use of diuretics or masking agents has become a covert biochemical science in direct competition with advances in methods of detection, a fact which marks the determination of some athletes to beat the system, and clearly points to a deliberate involvement of medical or paramedical persons in promoting the use of drugs in sport.

The other problem is that anabolic steroids, unlike β-blockers or short-term stimulants, are drugs primarily used during training for sporting events rather than at the time of competition. Since oral preparations are cleared from the body between two and 14 days after withdrawal, and injectables after a month, it is not difficult to use these agents during periods of intensive training and time their use so as to avoid detection at competitions. Thus detection would require random screening of athletes during training periods, a procedure for which few national sporting bodies have either the financial resources or the political will. Even were such testing to take place, it is unlikely that it would extend into body-building clubs, which remain largely immune because there are few competitions in which testing is carried out. This is in contrast to sports like athletics, swimming and Olympic weight-lifting, in which the Sports Council in this country spends £300000 a year on its drug-testing programme. Thus it remains difficult to see how elimination of the use of anabolic steroids can be achieved by this form of surveillance.

Is there a case against anabolic steroids?

Surprisingly, in the light of the above review, there is not unanimous agreement that anabolic steroids should be banned. The ethical issues are complex. Collier (1988) draws a parallel with use of the oral contraceptive pill by female athletes to ensure that menstruation does not occur during an important event. He states that 'the long-term health hazards from the oral contraceptive in women seem rather better documented that those for anabolic steroids taken by men'. This remains a fatuous conclusion, because of the much wider database from which the evidence on the oral contraceptive pill can be drawn, and because the secrecy surrounding information on the use of steroids in sport effectively conceals the denominator of the equation. Charles Yesalis, an epidemiologist at Pennsylvania State University, stated that 'we don't know what the long-term effects of steroid use are. The evidence linking them to liver and heart problems is extremely weak' (Cowart 1987). Certainly, long-term controlled studies might be necessary in order to produce firm 'scientific' evidence for the side-effects of steroids, and for the reasons already noted it is unlikely that these will ever take place. Cowart (1987) reports on the proposal to perform such a study in football players and power-lifters, but the protocol as reported seems deficient in a number of respects, not least in the omission of any form of liver scanning. In commenting on this study, Yesalis states 'I think we would have picked it up anecdotally by now if there were excess deaths in a group of young, healthy men'. I believe that the 'anecdotal' evidence for the adverse effects of steroids is adequate, and the only question that remains is whether banning the use of such preparations is ethically mandatory.

The pressures on certain types of sports men and women to use steroids in their training are considerable. At international competitive levels in power sports the use of any performance-enhancing drug may provide that critical 1 or 2% difference between victory and defeat, and the degree of drive and motivation at this level of competition is enormously high. In relation to professional sport, the pressures are economic as well as emotional. As John Lombardo of the Cleveland Clinic remarked 'a professional football player who is more than six feet tall and weighs 210 lbs might not make it to the pro ranks, whereas if he were stronger and weighed 240 lbs he might make $200 000 a year. As long as they are in that type of situation they will continue to use steroids'.

Howard Connelly, the 1956 Olymic hammer champion, said in 1973 'the overwhelming majority of athletes I know would do anything and take anything short of killing themselves to improve athletic performance'. It does now appear that a sufficiently determined athlete need not stop short of suicide in an attempt to win. Arguably, this is a matter for individual choice, and cannot ethically be restricted. However, it is this author's opinion that the inevitable transmission of such pressures to other athletes, and particularly down to young aspiring sports men and women, is more than enough ethical justification for continuing the ban on their use. How one achieves this objective remains a much more difficult issue.

References

Aiache A. E. (1989) Surgical treatment of gynecomastia in the bodybuilder. *Plastic and Reconstructive Surgery* **83**, 61–6.

Baltimore Evening Sun (1987) Harmful steroids trickle down to younger bodybuilders. June 8, p. 1.

Bernstein M. S., Hunter R. L. & Yachnin S. (1971) Hepatoma and peliosis hepatis developing in a patient with Fanconi's disease. *NEJM* **284**, 1135–6.

Bierly J. R. (1987) Use of anabolic steroids by athletes. Do the risks outweigh the benefits? *Postgraduate Medicine* **82**, 67–74.

BMJ News (1988) Anabolic steroids: the power and the glory? *BMJ* **297**, 877.

Catlin D. H., Kammerer R. C., Hatton C. K., Sekera M. H. & Merdink J. L. (1987) Analytical chemistry at the Games of the XXIIIrd Olympiad in Los Angeles, 1984. *Clinical Chemistry* **33**, 319–27.

Collier J. (1988) Drugs in sport: a counsel of perfection thwarted by reality. *British Medical Journal* **296**, 520.

Cowart V. S. (1987) Study proposes to examine football players, power lifters for possible long-term sequelae from anabolic steroid use in 1970s competition. *Journal of the American Medical Association* **257**, 3021–5.

Cowart V. S. (1989) Athlete drug testing receiving more attention than ever before in history of competition. *Journal of the American Medical Association* **261**, 3510–6.

Creagh T. M., Rubin A. & Evans D. J. (1988) Hepatic tumours induced by anabolic steroids in an athlete. *Journal of Clinical Pathology* **41**, 441–3.

Daily Telegraph (1987) Steroids blamed for body-builder's death, July 1.

Frankle M. A., Eichberg R. & Zachariah S. B. (1988) Anabolic androgenic steroids and a stroke in an athlete: case report. *Archives of Physical Medicine and Metabolism* **69**, 632–3.

Hamilton D. (1986) *The Monkey Gland Affair*. London: Chato & Windus.

Hatton C. K. & Catlin D. H. (1987) Detection of androgenic anabolic steroids in urine. *Clinics in Laboratory Medicine* **7**, 655–68.

Haupt H. A. & Rovere G. D. (1984) Anabolic steroids: a review of the literature. *American Journal of Sports Medicine* **12**, 469–84.

Kiraly C. L., Alen M., Rahkila P. & Horsmanheimo M. (1987) Effect of androgenic and anabolic steroids on the sebaceous gland in power athletes. *Acta Dermato-Venereologica* **67**, 36–40.

Krowchuk D. P., Anglin T. M., Goodfellow D. B., Stancin T., Williams P. & Zimet G. D. (1989) High school athletes and the use of ergogenic aid. *American Journal of Diseases of Children* **143**, 486–9.

Lamb, D. R. (1984) Anabolic steroids in athletics: how well do they work and how dangerous are they? *American Journal of Sports Medicine* **12**, 31–8.

Lenders J. W., Demacker P. N., Vos J. A., Jansen P. L., Hoitsma A. J., Van-t-Laar A. & Thien T. (1988) Deleterious effects of anabolic steroids on serum lipoproteins, blood pressure, and liver function in amateur bodybuilders. *International Journal of Sports Medicine* **9**, 19–23.

Lombardo J. (1987). Medical news and perspectives. *Journal of the American Medical Association* **257**, 3025.

McKillop G. (1987) Drug abuse in bodybuilders in the West of Scotland. *Scottish Medical Journal* **32**, 39–41.

McNutt R. A., Ferenchick G. S., Kirlin P. C. & Hamlin N. J. (1988) Acute myocardial infarction in a 22 year old world class weight lifter using anabolic steroids. *American Journal of Cardiology* **62**, 164.

Overly W. L., Dankoff J. A., Wang B. K. & Singh U. D. (1984) Androgens and hepatocellular carcinoma in an athlete. *Annals of Internal Medicine* **100**, 158–9.

Recant L. & Lacey P. (1965) Fanconi's anemia and hepatic cirrhosis. *American Journal of Medicine* **39**, 464.

Roberts J. T. & Essenhigh D. M. (1986) Adenocarcinoma of prostate in 40 year old bodybuilder (letter). *Lancet* **2**, 742.

Rosenbloom D. & Sutton J. R. (1985) Drugs and exercise. *Medical Clinics of North America* **69**, 177–87.

Stromeyer F. W., Smith D. H. & Ishak K. G. (1979) Anabolic steroid therapy and intrahepatic cholangiocarcinoma. *Cancer* **43**, 440–3.

Sweeney E. C. & Evans D. J. (1976) Hepatic lesions in patients treated with synthetic anabolic steroids. *Journal of Clinical Pathology* **29**, 626–33.

Westaby S., Portmann B. & Williams R. (1983) Androgen-related primary hepatic tumours in non-Fanconi patients. *Cancer* **51**, 1947–52.

Wright H. A. J. (1987) Medical news and perspectives. *Journal of the American Medical Association* **257**, 3025.

8 HIV disease and sport

C. LOVEDAY

'*Venienci occurite Morobo*' (meet the disease as it approaches)
Aulus Persius Flaccus

Human immunodeficiency virus (HIV) disease is a chronic retroviral
infection of human T-helper lymphocytes resulting in the gradual
but remorseless destruction of the immune system. Acute infection

Table 8.1 Cases of acquired immunodeficiency syndrome (AIDS) reported world-wide up to 31 March 1988

Continent	Country with more than 250 cases	Number of AIDS cases[a,c]
Africa[b]		10 995
	Burundi	960
	Central African Republic	254
	Congo	1 250
	Kenya	964
	Malawi	583
	Rwanda	901
	Tanzania	2 369
	Uganda	1 608
	Zaïre	335
	Zambia	536
	Zimbabwe	380
Americas		62 536
	Brazil	2 325
	Canada	1 517
	Dominican Republic	352
	Haiti	912
	Mexico	713
	USA	55 167
Asia		231
Europe		10 677
	Belgium	297
	Denmark	251
	France	3 073
	Holland	420
	Italy	1 619
	Spain	789
	Switzerland	355
	UK	1 344
	West Germany	1 848
Oceania		834
	Australia	758

[a] HIV antibody-positive individuals are 30–50 times this number.
[b] Actual cases very much higher as early cases are unrecognised, and case reporting is probably still not accurate.
[c] At time of going to press in September 1989 all numbers have doubled.

136

with HIV is followed by many years of chronic infection with no symptoms and few signs. As the disease progresses there is evidence of moderate immunodeficiency with recurrent common infections having an altered natural history and associated with constitutional symptoms and signs. End-stage disease, acquired immunodeficiency syndrome (AIDS), presents with opportunistic infection, unusual tumours and evidence of severe immunodeficiency.

Most acute HIV infections occur without symptoms. Development of anti-HIV antibodies occurs 4–12 weeks after infection and persists for life. Virus may be found in most body fluids but concentrations are highest in blood, semen and cervical secretions. Evidence suggests viral antigenaemia may fluctuate, being high early and late in the course of the disease with additional episodes of antigenaemia during the long asymptomatic phase of infection; thus it is probable that in individual's infectivity is variable and difficult to predict.

One hundred and thirty-three countries in the world have now reported cases of AIDS (85 273 March 1988) and it is certain there must exist an even larger unidentified population (30–50 times the AIDS cases) of asymptomatic HIV antibody-positive individuals (5–10 million world-wide) capable of transmitting the virus (Table 8.1).

Epidemiological data indicate that infection is spread by sexual contact and percutaneous and transplacental routes. Early in the epidemic high-risk groups (homosexual/bisexual men, intravenous drug users, haemophiliacs, transfusion recipients, prostitutes and sexual partners of all these) were identified, but infection has now spread outside these groups into the heterosexual population and it is no longer possible to predict reliably those who may be at risk.

At present there is no cure or vaccine available to treat the disease. Education is the only measure available to control the spread of infection.

Risk to sports competitors

Sports people, like any other individuals, are subject to general risks of infection by HIV, the greatest risk being that of sexual transmission. Thus, it is important that the number of sexual partners should be restricted and condoms used, especially when visiting countries where there is a high prevalence of HIV disease in the male and female populations (Table 8.1). The sharing of facilities (changing-rooms, showers, toilets, etc.), normal social contact and swimming pools constitute no danger of infection. Sharing of towels, razors, toothbrushes and 'bucket and sponge'* is a source of potential risk of all infections and should be discouraged.

---

*The 'bucket and sponge' communally used to 'treat' injuries in a wide variety of team sports must now be viewed as a mode of transmission of the virus, especially where bleeding has occurred. Sensible medical advice must therefore discourage the use of this traditional item of equipment and ban its use completely in areas of high risk (see Table 8.1).

Medical facilities in developing countries may not be presumed to be equivalent to those in the UK, and where HIV disease is prevalent must pose a further potential risk of infection. For sports people travelling and competing in such countries, 'immediate care packs', including sterile needles, syringes and intravenous fluids (blood substitutes), are available to take from the UK.

There is no documented evidence that contact sports (rugby, judo, etc.) have resulted in the transmission of HIV infection, but this area merits special consideration. HIV does not survive long in the open but there are a few documented cases of seroconversion following infected blood coming into contact with open skin lesions. With relatively low numbers of infected cases so far in existence, lesser modes of transmission may not be in evidence from epidemiological studies, but theoretically it must be conceded that a bleeding skin wound on an HIV-infected person must pose a risk to an opponent, in the event that infected blood comes into contact with or rubs against an open lesion on the skin of the uninfected opponent. If this (theoretical) risk becomes a reality considerable difficulties will exist for 'contact' sports in the future unless the HIV status of competitors is known. Such an undertaking is not without its own problems, e.g. who organises testing? is it mandatory? are individuals counselled? how often should individuals be tested?*

*This is an entirely new problem for the world of sporting activity and, in due course, must be addressed by individual governing bodies of respective sports which are at greatest risk.

Clearly these will relate to activities in which there is significant potential for blood loss in one or more of the participants, and will be especially concerned with whether a bleeding participant may continue to play and therefore run the risk of making direct physical contact with another player or players. Where blood from an infected player is spilt on to an open wound of another player there exists the risk of transmission of the virus. The necessity for precautions to eliminate this risk of cross-infection will naturally depend on the prevalence of the disease amongst participants. In parts of the world where significant numbers of the population are affected it would be prudent to advise sports men and women of the individual risks that they run. Players known to be positive should perhaps be excluded from selection and players who suffer significant wounds during play should either have these covered or be excluded from further participation. Preactivity testing for HIV status is fraught with legal and ethical problems and is probably not a practical proposition. However, if thought to be desirable, it should be coupled with full medical counselling of the implications of having the test.

Risk to first-aid workers, sports marshals and stewards

Many sporting activities involve the possibility of trauma and the resulting injuries pose risks to those who deliver immediate care to the competitors. The risks of HIV transmission in this setting may be put into perspective by considering the cases of occupationally acquired HIV disease so far documented. World-wide, a small number of cases of health-care workers infected during their work have been reported. These include: a female nurse in the UK who sustained a needlestick injury inoculation of approximately 1 ml of patient's blood, a female nurse in the USA receiving a deep intra-muscular needlestick injury, a female nurse from Martinique who sustained a needlestick injury without injection, a female nurse from France who sustained a superficial needlestick injury during thoracocentesis, a female nurse working ungloved with chapped skin whose hand was in contact with a patient's blood for 20 minutes during a cardiac arrest, a female phlebotomist with severe acne having blood splashed in her face, a female technologist who spilled contaminated blood on to her ungloved hands while carrying out plasmapheresis, and a male surgeon following work in Africa. Weighed against these cases are the results of follow-up studies of thousands of health-care workers who have had accidental contact with infected blood (Table 8.2), and only two seroconversions are documented here after at least one year's follow-up.

Thus the risks to those with unbroken skin coming in contact with infected blood are very small but do exist. These risks may be reduced further by the following recommended precautions:

1 Assume all casualties are HIV antibody-positive (never try to predict who may be positive).

2 Wear gloves for all procedures that involve contact with blood or other body secretions.

3 Cover all cuts or abrasions on hands with dressings before going on duty.

4 Wear glasses for procedures when blood may be splashed into the face.

5 Wash skin immediately after contamination with patient's blood or secretions.

6 Dispose of potentially infectious sharps safely; never attempt to resheathe needles.

	Number of staff	Type of exposure	Seroconversions at one year
Center for Disease Control, Atlanta, USA	1097	Needlestick, sharps, splash	1
National Institute of Health, USA	332	Needlestick	0
University of California, USA	63	Needlestick	0
Thames Health Regions, UK	150	Needlestick, sharps, splash	1

Table 8.2
Outcome of some studies of health-care workers exposed to HIV-infected blood

7   Dispose of waste materials by burning.

8   Clothing soiled with blood or secretions should be washed in a hot-cycle washing-machine, with a presoak for 30 minutes in hot soapy water at 70°C. If clothes cannot withstand these temperatures they can be soaked for 30 minutes in household bleach (1 in 10) or Milton solution diluted according to instructions.

9   Any other equipment or surfaces contaminated with blood may be treated with household bleach (as above).

10   Generally maintain sensible standards of hygiene.

11   Communal items such as a bucket and sponge have no further place in the care of injured sports people.

No cases of HIV infection resulting from mouth-to-mouth resuscitation have been described, but nevertheless it is recommended that one of the simple devices that are available for carrying out mouth-to-mouth ventilation (Table 8.3) with no direct contact between operator and patient is provided for use (i.e. carried by every first-aid worker or available at every marshal/first-aid post at sporting events).

It is essential that training programmes for all personnel are available to educate about risks of HIV infection and how to avoid them, and these should be repeated at intervals to ensure knowledge is up to date and to reduce complacency.

Summary

1   Sports people generally have the same risks of infection as the general population.

2   Certain contact sports pose a theoretically higher risk of virus transmission from one competitor to another. These risks are proportional to the prevalence to HIV-infected individuals in a given population, which varies markedly from country to country (see Table 8.1).

Table 8.3
Devices to assist in
mouth-to-mouth
ventilation

Laerdal pocket mask	Laerdal Medical, Stavanger, Norway
Sussex valve airway	Tandisdale Medical, Forest Row, Sussex, UK
Brook airway	G. H. Wood, Toronto, Canada
Resusciade	Portex Ltd, Hythe, Kent, UK
Sealeasy/Venteasy mask–airway	Respironus, Monroville, PA 15146N, USA
Dual aid	Vitalograph Ltd, Buckingham, UK

3   Potential risk of infection of first-aid workers, sports marshals and stewards is small but does exist. However, these risks can be reduced further by carrying out routine recommended precautions when caring for the injured.

9 The nature and incidence of injury in sport

J. G. P. WILLIAMS

'I have nothing to offer but blood, toil, tears and sweat'
Winston Churchill

Understanding injury

The major problems confronted in dealing with injuries due to accidents in sport lie in a common lack of understanding of the nature of such injuries. There are generally speaking no such things as football injuries or rugby injuries or athletics injuries — only injuries! Respective sports, however, will have their own well-recognized patterns of damage and special requirements of the participants, usually involving an early return to activity.

Injury is damage to the body caused by a mechanical stress to which it cannot adapt in time or space. When confronted by such a stress the body essays to adapt by avoidance, transmission or absorption. When none of these is possible, either because the intensity of the stress is too great or because the duration is too prolonged, damage occurs. The nature of the primary damage is dependent on the type of stress applied. The body is able to 'distinguish' between different mechanisms of stress (for example, a direct blow, as opposed to a sudden stretch) and this is reflected in the consequent tissue damage (Fig. 9.1), but it cannot differentiate between the different situations in which such a stress may be imposed (for example, in a road traffic accident, in a domestic accident or on the sports field).

The type of activity in which the victim is engaged at the time of the injury will, however, largely influence secondary features of the pathological response. For example, in the case of a fracture of the tibia and fibula haemorrhage will be far greater in a footballer who sustains his injury in the middle of an active game than in the case of a sedentary passenger similarly injured in a motor-car accident.

Physical fitness developed for participation in sport not only influences the secondary effects of injury but also significantly affects the recovery process therefrom. A haematoma may be very much bigger in an athlete with high blood flow through exercising limbs, but the very process of training prepares the limb for the rapid reabsorption of extravasated fluid, and therefore haematomas are more rapidly absorbed in fit, athletic individuals than in sedentary people. The essential similarity, in terms of tissue damage, of

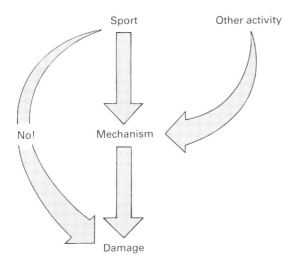

Sport   Other activity

No!   Mechanism

Damage

Fig. 9.1 Causal chain in injury.

the effects of similar stresses is particularly true in cases of in-stantaneous injury where relatively great external forces are applied, causing well-recognised damage patterns.

Problems, however, may arise in respect of overuse injuries (Corrigan 1968). These are due to internal stresses generated chronically during training and are relatively uncommon outside the sporting context, although they may be observed in the enthusiastic 'do-it-yourselfer' who suddenly engages in unaccustomed activity. They also occur in some areas of industry involving people who take up new jobs requiring unaccustomed repetitive activity, and they may also be met in 'high-performance' occupations, for example the armed forces, where the development of high levels of physical fitness are required. Until recently the aetiology, pathology and incidence of overuse injury were relatively uncertain, but there has been wide documentation of such injuries and a considerable litera-ture in the English language is readily available (Williams & Sperryn 1976; O'Donoghue 1984; Helal *et al.* 1986).

In addition to specific injuries patients may present with clinical problems due less to specific stress overload than to secondary condi-tions, usually constitutional, which lead to biomechanical inad-equacies for the activity performed, thus enhancing and multiplying the effect of what, for a normal person, would be acceptable stress levels. Examples include long-distance runners and joggers who have torsion of the tibia and excessively pronating feet, which on a day-to-day basis may cause no problems. Under the stresses of running or jogging, however, the faulty biomechanics makes the absorption of otherwise reasonable stress levels impossible, and breakdown occurs.

An important factor in injury in sport is that frequently symp-toms and signs may be vague because presentation occurs in earlier states of the condition. In the trained, high-performance individual,

144
Chapter 9
The nature and
incidence of
injury in sport

whether in sport or in any other physical activity, a relatively minor problem in clinical terms can cause significant and considerable disability. Most patients in ordinary, mildly active or sedentary lives can cope readily with injuries, whether of the impact or over-use type, that would significantly and adversely affect the performance of an active sports man or woman of élite class.

Although symptoms and signs on presentation may be relatively diffuse and difficult to interpret, they must not be taken lightly. It is salutary to note the frequency with which significant and serious pathology first presents as discomfort of a vague, and initially mild, nature associated with physical activity, particularly sport. There are many recorded instances, for example, of osteomyelitis and bone tumours making their first presentation in athletes as vague pain during exercise (Williams 1980). The nature of these symptoms is explained by pressure effects associated with hyperaemia of exercise. It is important for the attending clinician to make every effort to reach an accurate diagnosis and to be aware of the usual natural history of the condition diagnosed. Any variation from the familiar pattern of disease diagnosed should arouse suspicion and indicate the need for careful investigation.

Further complications arise when real injury occurs in pathological tissue. The case is recorded of an athlete who experienced sudden pain in the quadriceps muscle during training. On the face of it, this was a straightforward rectus femoris tear. There was no previous history. Clinically the patient had considerable swelling and bruising of the quadriceps with a tender mass in the front of the thigh. He was treated as a muscle tear and showed initially a good response. Subsequently, however, the swelling recurred without pain and the lesion proved to be a rhabdomyosarcoma. It was later demonstrated that there had been haemorrhage into the tumour mass and the muscle rupture had been of the sarcomatous rather than the normal muscle tissue. For such a lesion, however, it would be virtually impossible and probably undesirable to submit all patients with apparent muscle tears to ultrasound or computerised tomography (CT) scanning in order to detect rare malignancy. Cases of this sort nevertheless emphasise that things may not always be as they seem. The attending clinician must always maintain a degree of suspicion and at least be aware of the extent to which serious pathology may present as relatively innocuous injury.[*]

The vast majority of injuries in sport do not require any form of specialised knowledge or treatment. Even in a selected series attending specialist sports injuries clinics it has been shown that

---

[*] In the case described failure to detect the sarcoma at first presentation would be unlikely to be construed as negligence, on account of the rarity of the condition and the presence of another reasonable explanation for the presenting symptoms. The importance of careful follow-up for apparently innocuous conditions is, however, well demonstrated.

145
Chapter 9
The nature and
incidence of
injury in sport

more than 60% of cases could have been dealt with perfectly well by the patient's family doctor or by a recognised specialist in loco-motor disorders (Sperryn & Williams 1975). Across the population of sport men and women as a whole, the percentage of patients re-quiring highly specialist sports medical experience is substantially lower.

However, it must be remembered that a knowledge and under-standing of the mechanics of injury in sport and its specialist man-agement can only be acquired by formal study. Specific instruc-tion in the peculiar problems of injured sports men and women should be obtained by doctors who seek to pursue a career in sports medicine.

One major difficulty facing the interested clinician is the plethora of anecdotal and otherwise unreliable material disseminated in both printed and verbal form. This has led inevitably to the encourage-ment and practice of ideas and treatment measures which do not always stand up to close inspection. Amongst these may be included the use of steroids by injection, the use of therapeutic ultrasound and even the use of cold for treatment. All these modalities of treat-ment are popular in the management of sports injuries, and all carry a significant element of risk. One of the depressing features of sports medical practice is the frequency with which patients present with iatrogenic problems related to the use of these and other forms of treatment.

Classification of injury in sport

Injuries in sport can be classified in a number of ways (Williams 1971). Classification by aetiology or causation is useful in that it assists in reaching the diagnosis through an appreciation of the mechanism of injury.

Essentially athletes and sports men and women present either with injuries sustained during sport which usually prevent further participation or alternatively with injuries sustained incidentally to the sports activity but which also interfere with subsequent par-ticipation. In the latter case injuries exist in a similar spectrum to those encountered in the population at large.

Injuries occurring in sport may be primary, that is to say the direct result of a specific stress or overload, or secondary, where the pathological condition has been itself provoked by some previous injury. For example, the anterior knee pain syndrome (chondroma-lacia patellae) may be secondary to some previous relatively minor knee injury which has caused quadriceps inhibition, which, through muscle imbalance, has in turn provoked the development of chon-dromalacia. Many causes of spinal pain, particularly in the low back, derive as secondary lesions from some previous relatively minor insult.

146

Chapter 9
The nature and
incidence of
injury in sport

King (1983) has also described a 'second injury' phenomenon. It occurs when an athlete or sports man or woman sustains a minor injury and continues to play instead of resting, thereby making himself/herself vulnerable to a second unrelated, but possibly more severe, injury.

Primary injury may derive either from forces generated outside the patient's body, in which case they are referred to as extrinsic, or from forces generated within, when they are described as intrinsic. Extrinsic injuries are usually instantaneous and cause more severe damage than intrinsic injury, because the mechanical forces involved are greater. Many of these injuries are similar to impact injuries in other activities, for example, dislocation of the shoulder occurs with monotonous regularity in rugby football as it does in domestic accidents. Various factors have been recognised in contributing to extrinsic injury, these being human, implemental, vehicular and environmental.

Intrinsic injuries derive specifically from the patient's own activities and may occur in a single incident or, more commonly, as a result of repeated stress overload. Single-incident injuries include sudden, complete rupture of the Achilles tendon, or a hamstring tear, whereas overuse injuries involve compartment syndromes, tendinitis and stress fractures.

As in all cases of injury, a carefully taken history should indicate the nature of the problem, particularly where there is adequate background knowledge of the natural history of the injury and of the mechanics of the sport. A common error of diagnosis — due specifically to lack of knowledge of its natural history — is misdiagnosis of sciatica as 'chronic hamstring strain', which occurs all too frequently. Pain, initially of gradual onset, experienced in the back of the thigh is not due to a 'pulled' muscle. A muscle tear occurs instantaneously and the onset of pain is therefore sudden. Gradual onset of pain in the back of the thigh during exercise is almost invariably sciatica, due to lumbar nerve root irritation. Too often practitioners, unaware of this simple fact, misdiagnose sciatica and patients are then subjected to more or less protracted periods of completely ineffective treatment directed to the hamstrings instead of to the primary cause in the lumbar spine.

Patterns of injury in sport

While it is true that there are no 'sport-specific' injuries as such, it is nevertheless possible to discern regular patterns of injury in different types of sport which are related to the mechanisms of stress within those sports (Weightman & Browne 1974). Indeed there may be changes in the patterns of injury within a given sport as a result of changes in the way that the sport is practised, often due to changes in the laws and regulations which govern it. In Rugby

147

Chapter 9
The nature and
incidence of
injury in sport

Union football, for example, there has been a reduction, both real and relative, in the incidence of cervical injuries as a result of changes in the laws relating to the scrummage (Burry & Calcinai 1988; see also Chapter 3). A further redefinition of the laws of this phase of the game would probably diminish further the risks of such injuries. At the same time there appears to be an increase in other types of contact injuries in rugby, in part caused by the practice of 'hyping up' teams before playing, so raising unnecessarily the level of aggression. The margin between what is fair and what is unfair and improper thus becomes progressively blurred. It is interesting to note that in rugby football 30% of injuries occur in a 'foul' situation (Davies & Gibson 1978).*

Patterns that may be clearly discerned across the whole spectrum of sports show that in Rugby Union and the other codes of football, in addition to judo, wrestling and boxing and indeed all 'body-contact sports', direct impact injuries are more common than in tennis or track and field athletics. Players in racket sports tend to have an increased frequency of injuries affecting the upper limbs, while track athletes show different patterns of injury according to the type of event in which they are competing. Sprinters, for example, tend to have upper leg injuries, whereas in middle- and long-distance runners injuries tend to affect the lower leg.

It is tempting to classify injuries according to the sport, but this may be counter-productive in the sense that this tends to encourage fixed ideas as to what may or may not occur in a given sport. This often leads to conditions being missed because they were not regarded as being characteristic of the sport in question. What is needed in order to understand injury is a clear conception of its mechanism. Frequently the diagnosis becomes immediately apparent from the description of the way in which the injury occurred. Thus, for example, the football player who complains of pain and instability in the knee following an incident in which this foot was held in the ground by the studs of his boot while his body turned away from the knee, which was flexed, weight-bearing, abducted and externally rotated, would almost certainly have developed anteromedial rotary instability with damage to the medial meniscus and collateral ligament, capsule and possibly the anterior cruciate ligament. Given an accurate description from the patient himself or herself or from reliable witnesses as to how the accident occurred, the diagnosis usually becomes clear. To some extent this is also the case in an overuse injury; a clear description of the

---

* This to an extent may be something of a self-fulfilling prophecy, for the referee as the sole judge of fact on the field of play decides what is and is not 'foul play'. There remains scope, however, to further reduce the incidence of injuries during play by further alteration of the rules to avoid potentially dangerous situations, e.g. the 'pile-up', and by attempting to influence referees to become more discerning in distinguishing between legitimate enthusiasm and aggression constituting foul play.

148

Chapter 9
The nature and
incidence of
injury in sport

patient's training programme will often give a strong clue as to what is going wrong.

In the same way that a sound grasp of fundamental anatomy and biomechanics is required for the proper interpretation of case histories of injured sports men and women, so too is an understanding of the nature of the sport in question valuable. This is not to say that it is a prerequisite that the practitioner should necessarily have any specific experience of the sport. It is advantageous, however, to be able to interpret accurately the player's description of that phase of the game in which he was injured, and to this end it is useful but not essential to have at least a working knowledge of the rules and method of play.

In many instances injuries occur as a result of faulty technique, particularly in highly technical events (such as hammer-throwing), and correction of technique becomes an essential component of patient management. This is particularly so in a situation where as a result of injury the patient has developed bad habits. It is not necessarily every practitioner of sports medicine who is in a position to advise and coach patients out of their technical faults — but it is open to all to make certain that the patient is referred to a suitable authority in the sport for expert guidance for fault correction to prevent recurrence.

An important practical problem for the practitioner relates to the return of the patient to training and competition, particularly the latter. It is often said that the athletic patient 'wants to be 110% fit and he wants it yesterday'. Many athletes and sports men and women, particularly in the professional ranks, are often under severe pressure to return to sporting activity too soon. A major disadvantage of the system (in association football for example) of allowing substitutes on to the field is the temptation, to which managers frequently yield, of putting in a player who is far from fully fit, because the player in question has a considerable drawing power in terms of the number of spectators (and the financial benefits to the club accruing therefrom).*

There is in the pressure of the sporting situation a considerable temptation to take risks and cut corners in treatment so as to allow an undesirably rapid resumption of sporting activity. It is possible that in certain circumstances (particularly where the administration of drugs of one kind or another may be concerned) the practitioner may be pressurised into so inappropriate an attempt to restore the sports man or woman to competition that this may later be regarded as malpractice for which the practitioner might

---

* For the medical practitioner asked to advise in this situation, a dilemma may arise. The relationship between the doctor and the club is usually that the doctor is an agent of the club, receiving financial or other material reward for his services. The discharge of his duties toward the club, therefore, may conflict with the best interests of the 'patients'.

be held liable for negligence (Ford 1980). There are times when the sports doctor finds himself walking a moral tightrope. It is important, therefore, that these issues should have been considered by the doctor, that he keeps good notes and that he feels confident that he would be able to justify his actions if subsequently challenged.

149

Chapter 9
The nature and
incidence of
injury in sport

Misdiagnosis of injury

Until quite recently, and still in some instances today, sport as a human activity has been viewed with disfavour by medical practitioners. Patients who become injured in such activities thus often receive scant attention or sympathy from family doctors or hospital practitioners. Such an uncaring attitude invariably prejudices correct history-taking and a proper and careful examination. The attitude 'go away and rest it and don't bother me' is still too prevalent and may lead to disaster. Examples are regularly met of infection and tumours which first presented as pain in sport and have been left undiagnosed for too long because of a negative attitude to active treatment by the practitioner concerned. (Such attitudes and simple lack of care can of course be met in a variety of situations and do not always apply to sports men and women.)

Two clinical traps which have medico-legal implications and which occur commonly in sports men and women and non-sports men and women alike are the undiagnosed fracture of the waist of the scaphoid and the undiagnosed slipped upper femoral epiphysis (Hawkins 1985). These conditions are regularly featured in the annual reports published by the Medical Protection Society, and cautionary tales too often go unheeded.

Ignorance is perhaps the main reason why crises arise in the management of sports injuries. Most practitioners are able to deal effectively with major trauma, but apparently minor, yet nevertheless disabling, conditions remain inadequately diagnosed and treated.

There is an extensive and often excellent literature available at a variety of academic levels covering the whole spectrum of injury in sport, particularly those injuries which are not part of common orthopaedic or trauma practice. It is therefore remarkable how often these texts are unheeded (or perhaps not understood!) and even quite obvious pathologies misdiagnosed and consequently mistreated. One such example is complete rupture of the Achilles tendon (Medical Defence Union 1977). There should never be any difficulty in accurate diagnosis of this condition, yet it is frequently missed, patients being referred to physiotherapists for muscle strain. The condition is relatively uncommon but nevertheless should be familiar to general practitioners and accident and emergency department doctors.

150

Chapter 9
The nature and
incidence of
injury in sport

Mismanagement of injury

Over past years a plethora of new types of physical treatment has been introduced, the biological effects of some of which are still uncertain. Such methods of treatment are sometimes used with a worrying lack of discernment by various practitioners, particularly physiotherapists.

Ultrasound therapy is commonly used for soft tissue injuries without scientific measurement of the dose delivered or its direction. The therapist may have some idea of the output from the sound-head but has no means of determining the dose at tissue level or its biological effects. Studies by Dyson and others (Dyson *et al.* 1974; Dyson 1985) have indicated the type and extent of damage that treatment of this type may cause, yet it is still used in a rather haphazard fashion by practitioners who have only the sketchiest idea of its effects. Its value in some cases has been well established (Binder *et al.* 1985), but the number of clinical trials of this and other forms of physiotherapy that can be regarded as sound is very small. Histological examination, particularly of the ultrastructure of tendon material removed at surgery for chronic Achilles tendon pain, has indicated a significant degree of damage to the tendon. This accords remarkably closely with the damage observed by Dyson in experimental studies of tissues which had received excessive insonation. It may be that many cases of persistent Achilles tendon pain are partially iatrogenic in that lesions are possibly made worse by excessive insonation.

Another form of treatment in common use for sports injuries is cold, in the form of cold water baths, the application of a bag of frozen peas, endothermic commercial compresses and simple ice-bags. The risk to the integrity of the peripheral nerves in areas of cooling has been clearly defined (Bickford 1939; Pamchenko 1944). Furthermore, many patients show evidence of prolonged impairment of function after treatment with cold. It is dubious, therefore, whether such treatment specifically and favourably influences many of the conditions for which it is used, for example, ankle sprains or muscle tears.

The use of these treatment modalities has been hallowed, perhaps incorrectly, by years of practice without critical reappraisal. The sporting public's heightened expectations in respect of proper medical management may in future prove to be just the required stimulus to proper critical appraisal of methods of treatment currently in vogue which are popular without being rational.

Another form of treatment frequently but sometimes injudiciously practised by doctors and others is injection of local anaesthetic and steroid. The full effects of this type of treatment are also uncertain. There are many instances recorded in the literature of damage caused by such injections both in experimental and in therapeutic

151

Chapter 9
The nature and
incidence of
injury in sport

models (Ismail *et al.* 1969; Unverferth & Olix 1973; Kennedy & Baxter Willis 1976). The classic, perhaps, is complete rupture of the Achilles tendon following steroid injection for tendinitis. Ruptures can also occur at other sites, in addition to areas of scar breakdown and other pathological changes in injected tissues. Steroid stigmata including loss of subcutaneous fat, discoloration and scar stretching are well recognised and frequently seen in sports patients.

'Prevention is better than cure'

It has ever been the lesson of the Medical Protection Society and its sister organisations that prevention is better than cure. Prevention of unnecessary injury and damage in sports men and women demands a proper knowledge of sports traumatology and its correct application. The practice of sports medicine requires the same elements of care, dedication and study as any other branch of medicine.

References

Bickford R. G. (1939) The fibre dissociation produced by cooling human nerves. *Clinical Science* **4**, 159–65.

Binder A., Hodge G., Greenwood A. M., Hazleman B. L. & Page-Thomas D. P. (1985) Is therapeutic ultrasound effective in treating soft tissue lesions? *British Medical Journal* **290**, 512.

Burry H. C. & Calcinai C. J. (1988) The need to make rugby safer. *British Medical Journal* **296**, 149–50.

Corrigan A. B. (1968) Sports injuries. *Hospital Medicine* **2**, 1328–34.

Davies J. E. & Gibson T. (1978) Injuries in Rugby Union football. *British Medical Journal* **2** (6154), 1759–61.

Dyson M. (1985) Therapeutic applications of ultrasound. In *Clinics in Diagnostic Ultrasound*, vol. 16, *Biological Effects of Ultrasound*, ed. W. L. Nyborg & M. C. Ziskin, pp. 121–33. New York: Churchill Livingstone.

Dyson M., Bond J. B., Woodward B. & Broadhurst J. (1974) The production of blood all stasis and endothelial damage in the blood vessels of chick embryos treated with ultrasound in a stationary wave field. *Ultrasound in Medicine and Biology* **1**, 133–48.

Ford P. G. T. (1980) Ethics in sports medicine — some medico-legal considerations. *British Journal of Sports Medicine* **14**, 90–1.

Hawkins C. (1985) *Mishap or Malpractice?* Oxford: Blackwell Scientific Publications.

Helal B., King J. B. & Grange W. J. (1986) *Sports Injuries and their Treatment*. London: Chapman & Hall.

Ismail A. M., Balakrishnan R. & Rajakumar M. K. (1969) Rupture of patellar ligament after steroid infiltration. *Journal of Bone Joint Surgery* **51B**, 503–5.

Kennedy J. C. & Baxter Willis R. (1976) The effects of local injection of steroids into tendons — a biomechanical and microscopic study. *American Journal of Sports Medicine* **4**, 11–21.

King J. B. (1983) Second injury syndrome (Letter). *British Journal of Sports Medicine* **17**, 59–60.

Medical Defence union (1977) *Annual Report 1977*. London: Medical Defence Union.

O'Donoghue D. H. (1984) *Treatment of Injuries to Athletes*, 4th edn. Philadelphia: W. B. Saunders.

Pamchenko D. I. (1944) Retrograde changes in the spinal cord in frost bite of the extremities. *American Review of Soviet Medicine* **1**, 440–3.

Sperryn P. N. & Williams J. G. P. (1975) Why sports injuries clinics? *British Medical Journal* **3**, 364–5.

Unverferth L. J. & Olix M. L. (1973) The effect of local steroid injection on tendons. *Journal of Sports Medicine and Physical Fitness* **1** (4), 31–7.

Weightman D. & Browne R. C. (1974) Injuries in Association and Rugby Football. *British Journal of Sports Medicine* **8**, 183–7.

152

*Chapter 9
The nature and
incidence of
injury in sport*

Williams J.G.P. (1971) Aetiological classification of injury in sportsmen. *British Journal of Sports Medicine* **5**, 228–30.

Williams J.G.P. (1980) *A Colour Atlas of Injury in Sport*. London: Wolfe Medical.

Williams J.G.P. & Sperryn P.N. (1976) *Sports Medicine*, 2nd Edn. London: Edward Arnold.

The doctor's contribution towards safety in sport — an exercise in preventive medicine 10

D. A. D. MACLEOD

'Beneath the rule of men entirely great the pen is mightier than the sword'
From *Richelieu II*, ii, by E. C. Lytton

Prologue

The identification of risk factors and their eradication both for healthy living and in sport are exercises in preventive medicine. So much has been written about whether sports medicine really is a speciality or specialism. If one considers, however, the two main components of sports medicine — the physiological assessment of fitness or exercise medicine, and the prevention and treatment of injuries — then sports medicine, albeit dealing with a particular healthcare population, is in itself an exercise in preventive medicine.

In rugby union football, besides the identification of risk factors through epidemiological and clinical injury surveys, the structure of injury care is itself a challenge in preventive medicine.

Most rugby games, apart from senior international and representive matches, are unattended by doctors or physiotherapists. The grass roots matches in many parts of the country and the world are watched by one man and his dog, if that!

Two rugby playing countries have tried to overcome the problem of first-aid cover at matches, but both in different ways and for some different reasons. In Wales, with a playing population of over 30 000 each weekend, many games are attended by members of the Welsh Association of Sports Trainers. This is an association of members of the lay-public in general, who are given courses and lectures on sports first-aid, are given accreditation and who play an invaluable role in the primary care of the injured played. If necessary, the paramedical and medical professions are the second part of contact, and hospitalization and surgery are the third. This tripartite structure serves the rugby playing community well.

In Japan, where there are over 120 000 players each weekend, rugby players have the same problem as the Japanese golfers, an inadequate number of playing pitches. To counteract this logistical problem, there are some playing grounds throughout Japan where several matches are played on the same pitch on the same day, starting at 6.00 a.m. in the morning and continuing until the evening! As rugby is also played nearly all the year round, most of the playing surfaces are devoid of any grass. The Kento Medical Society in Japan is a society of over 300 rugby doctors who ensure that most of these pitches each have an ambulance, a doctor and

153

154

Chapter 10
The doctor's
contribution
towards safety in
sport

paramedical personnel in attendance throughout the day. The society consists mainly of primary care practitioners, orthopaedic surgeons and rehabilitationists, and hold annual conferences on rugby medicine.

One can always learn from other countries and other sports to introduce safety factors. In Sweden for instance, every sporting participant has to be licensed by the respective governing body to partake in that sport. The licence is linked to an accident and injury insurance scheme which is compulsory and is underwritten and insured by one company only, Folksam. This company, through their computerised programme, have statistics on all injuries in every sport and in turn provide information on risk areas to each governing body who may introduce legislation to make the sport safer.

The philosophy of the Scandinavian countries on the whole is similar to that in the UK with regard to the ethics of sport and fair play, and this also applies to the question of drugs in sport.

International rugby, through the World Cup and, at the time of writing, possible changes in the laws appertaining to amateurism, is facing its biggest challenge yet. Administrators and the rugby medical profession, by continual monitoring of risk factors in the game, epidemiological surveys and worldwide introduction of randomized dope testing, should ensure wherever possible that rugby keeps to the Olympic ideal of sportsmanship and fair play.

John E. Davies

All responsible governing bodies in sport should ensure that the common patterns of injury that are associated with their particular discipline are identified and minimised, wherever practical, by appropriate changes in the laws of the sport concerned. Any change in the laws under which a sport is conducted ought to be introduced with an appropriate educational programme involving participants, coaches and officials.

It is important not to lose sight of the fact that sport must at the same time retain its inherent challenge and character. These qualities lead inevitably to a degree of risk, which will be associated with a certain number of unavoidable injuries.

Exercise programmes designed to promote the physical well-being of individuals, irrespective of their age, should be structured in such a way that risk is minimal and the prospect of injury eliminated.

Individuals participate in sport for many different and complex reasons. The majority of sports men and women participate in sport to promote their physical fitness and for fun, enjoying the camaraderie of the event or the club to which they belong. This applies in both individual pursuits and team games. Inevitably there is an increased risk of injury in contact and collision sports, compared with individual activities and racket sports.

Many leisure activities which are undertaken on an individual and unsupervised basis such as hill-walking, horse-riding and swimming are associated with significant risks of both catastrophic and

155
*Chapter 10
The doctor's
contribution
towards safety in
sport*

minor injuries. The real dangers associated with these activities are constantly underestimated and this is particularly true with regard to hill-walking in the Scottish mountains, where approximately 20% of 'call-outs' of the Scottish Mountain Rescue Teams are to recover the dead (McGregor 1988).

Although most sports men and women pursue their pastime 'for fun' by comparison, a proportion of amateur sports men and women constantly strive to achieve greater and greater peaks of performance. Irrespective of the nature of the sport in which they are involved, there is an inevitable sharp increase in the risk of injury associated with increasing demands of training and competition when the athlete is striving to reach the very limits of his or her potential. It is well recognised that, the greater the number and intensity of training sessions and competitions undertaken by international athletes, the greater is the risk of injury in both amateur and professional sport. These injuries may be due to fatigue, physical stress, overuse, psychological burn-out or simply increased opportunities for damage. In professional sport, there is additional pressure on the athlete to 'perform', irrespective of any niggling minor injury or illness that may be present: 'No play — no pay'. The additional financial pressures placed on professional athletes to perform to entertain and to win are inevitably associated with very different attitudes towards their injuries and their sport.

Sport, whether it is undertaken for fitness, for fun, or as a profession, should not be associated with avoidable risks of injury or illness during either training or competition. Most athletes' active participation in sport, particularly if they are the élite striving for success or are professionals, tends to be relatively short-lived because of the physical and psychological demands placed upon them. Participation in sport at the top level in the twenties or early thirties age-groups should not inevitably mean permanent disability or premature ageing. The psychological stresses of retirement from sport are sufficiently distressing in themselves without having to face the additional burdens of disability that could have been avoided by appropriate training programmes and coaching techniques, as well as by education or sports legislation designed to minimise the risk of injury, and good medical care. Athletes striving for success should not be considered as experimental physiological preparations, and the pressures to which they are subjected by enthusiastic coaches and sports scientists should be monitored by appropriately trained and committed doctors.

Role and responsibilities of doctors

One of the significant problems that has deterred doctors from undertaking studies to identify the risks in association with sport is the difficulty in agreeing a definition of 'an injury'. There is no

156

Chapter 10
The doctor's
contribution
towards safety in
sport

difficulty with major injuries, but with minor and moderate injuries it can be extremely difficult to agree with both the athletes and the coaches involved in the sport under consideration. Many athletes would include impaired performance in the definition of an injury. Performance is linked to both psychological and physical factors. The same applies to a definition based on time lost from training; from this point of view the definition of an injury might relate to whether or not the athlete sought medical advice. Such a definition is not reliable, however, as it would also have to take into account the availability of a doctor for consultation at the time of perceived need. Many athletes prefer to take their injuries to a physiotherapist or other practitioners of alternative medicine.

It has been agreed in rugby football that studies undertaken to identify the causative factors resulting in injury should only include those injuries which prevent the player participating in the sport one week after the injury occurred, or if the player has been admitted to hospital. This definition eliminates many of the minor grazes, lacerations and bumps and bruises that are concomitant with collision sport and are assumed to be part of the ordinary risk of participating in rugby football.

In the future, it seems likely that increasing pressure will be placed on the governing bodies of sport as the number of participants in both leisure and sporting activities increases. With each succeeding generation, the population as a whole tends to get bigger and stronger. Training programmes and modern coaching techniques improve the overall fitness of athletes participating in sport at all levels, as well as changing the attitudes of athletes involved in an activity. In these circumstances, any governing body which fails to review the changing pattern of risk associated with their sport will lose the confidence of their participants. Equally, any law change produced by the governing body must be monitored closely from the point of view of safety to ensure that the hoped-for change which was sought by the alteration in laws is not associated with an increased risk of injury.

Increasing consumer sophistication among athletes and coaches will place increasing pressure on the medical profession to ensure that their knowledge of exercise physiology and sports medicine is of the highest standard. It is inevitable that doctors involved in sport will be subjected to continued monitoring of their standards of clinical practice. This will have to be associated with improved formal teaching programmes at both undergraduate and postgraduate level, examinations to monitor performance and the eventual development of a recognised speciality in exercise and sports medicine. This speciality would be equivalent in status to occupational health or accident and emergency medicine and surgery.

In 1987 the Scottish Sports Council published a short guide for governing bodies of sport on the provision of medical advisory services. In this guide, the Scottish Sports Council recommended that an effective medical service would identify, document and analyse risk factors associated with injury or illness in their sport, and then recommend appropriate measures that could be taken to minimise the risks. The medical team would have to possess a substantial knowledge of the sport in question and establish a close liaison with the participants, coaches, officials and administrators responsible for the designing of safe laws for that activity. The medical team will be expected to give advice about first-aid requirements for players. The medical team might also be involved in the development of safe and effective protective equipment for participants in the sport which could not in any way harm an opponent. The medical team would ensure that the environment in which the sport was undertaken was safe and practical, with, for example padded posts and, where appropriate, flexible non-shattering poles at goal-lines, for corner flags, etc. The playing surface and the immediate surrounds should not be cluttered with dangerous 'street furniture' such as advertising boardings and spectator barriers into which an athlete might accidentally crash. The medical team would have to clarify whether they were to undertake responsibility for the safety of spectators as well as players. Spectator safety presents vastly different problems and requires liaison with different agencies and emergency services (see Chapter 5).

Athletes participating in sport accept the obvious and foreseeable risks that might reasonably be associated with the activity in question, assuming that the event is undertaken within the rules, and that the rules have been designed to ensure fair and safe competition. Sporting behaviour by athletes would ensure that they honour these rules and respect both their opponent and the decisions of the officials. Unfortunately, in the present day and age, sporting behaviour has a tendency to be replaced by 'gamesmanship' and many athletes and coaches devote considerable time and energy to devising techniques which will overcome their opponents by playing to the limit of the rules and sometimes beyond. The presence of the doctor at training sessions as well as matches can help emphasise the importance of adopting safe techniques.

Doctors involved in sport have an ethical and legal duty to provide competent professional services and to ensure that they practise medicine to a high standard with appropriate facilities. The doctor has an additional ethical responsibility with regard to the prevention of injury by advising that appropriate protective equipment is worn by the players, the environment is safe, and vulnerable individuals do not participate in an event when there is a risk of aggravating a primary injury or sustaining a second, invariably more serious, injury. If a doctor recognises a pattern of events leading to injury, he has an ethical duty to draw this to the attention of the players, coaches and legislators, in the hope that this pattern can

157
*Chapter 10
The doctor's
contribution
towards safety in
sport*

158
Chapter 10
The doctor's
contribution
towards safety in
sport

be broken and the injuries minimised. On occasion, the doctor may be faced with a situation where an injury has resulted from violence outside the rules of the game. This may occur as a result of careless of thoughtless play, but may be the result of deliberate cheating, recklessness or violence and, in these circumstances, the doctor has a duty both to treat the injured player and to protect other players from similar violence by informed liaison with the relevant official in the event, club or sport and the individuals concerned.[*]

Minimising the dangers of sport

The player who elects to participate in a sport accepts the ordinary risks of this activity. In many sports, significant dangers do exist and all players must accept the responsibility of minimising serious injury. A resurgence of the old-fashioned concept of sporting behaviour, in which an athlete respected the opponent, played within the spirit and laws of the game, and honoured the officials, would go a long way towards making the life of sports legislators and the doctors involved in sport a lot easier.

American football

Many sports have made major achievements adopting the principles outlined above. In 1964, the American Association of Neurological Surgery initiated a series of studies into catastrophic injuries in American football. Over the subsequent years, detailed analysis of these catastrophic injuries, which included death and permanent paralysis, was undertaken. In 1968, 36 fatalities occurred in 1.25 million American football players. As a result of detailed cooperation and scientific research initiated by the medical profession in conjunction with American football coaches, a series of modifications to the laws, equipment and coaching techniques has achieved a dramatic improvement in the situation and only four catastrophes occurred in 1983. The achievements of the medical profession working with the governing bodies of American football make inspiring reading and are reviewed in detail in Schneider *et al* (1985).

Rugby

In 1978, the International Rugby Football Board established a Medical Advisory Committee to advise the board on the incidence of injuries occurring in Rugby Union with a view to identifying

[*]A conflict of interests between the doctor and his patient and the doctor and the controlling body arises here. This may be overcome by anonymous reporting of incidents or probably more practically by analysis and reporting of trends of injury coupled with suggested changes in the laws where appropriate.

relevant risk factors and modifying the laws of the game. Since that date, a number of major law changes in rugby union, in conjunction with a series of resolutions and recommendations, have been made on the basis of improving player safety. Among these changes are the following:

1 Elimination of the 'high tackle'.

2 Changes in the laws relating to scrummaging to improve the stability of the scrum, reduce the impact or collision forces as the scrum is formed, and penalise attempts to pull down or collapse the scrum. The range through which the scrum may rotate, has also been controlled by legislation.

3 Changes in the laws relating to the tackle, the ruck and the maul, encouraging quick release of the ball and ensuring that players stay on their feet.

4 International rugby has accepted the need for doping control to eliminate cheating by the taking of drugs. Rugby has, in addition, included in its recommendations a statement that players should not participate in rugby if they require drugs or injections for relief of acute illness or injury. Doping control in rugby includes testing for the presence of injectable local anaesthetic agents.

5 Detailed recommendations have been made with regard to the appropriate matching of players participating in rugby at school, during youth and at under-18 and under-21 levels, stressing the importance of assessing an individual player's maturity rather than solely judging his abilities on age.

6 The International Rugby Football Board has repeatedly advised players to purchase and use individually fitted dental mouth-guards to protect their teeth and reduce the risk of both orofacial and concussional head injuries.

7 The International Rugby Football Board has stressed the recommendation that any player who has been concussed should not participate in a rugby match for a minimum of three weeks after his head injury, and only when an appropriate medical examination has been undertaken.

Boxing

Boxing as a sport has been subject to considerable criticism by certain medical groups. Much work has been undertaken by the medical profession in assessing the damaging effects of both amateur and professional boxing and the consequences or cumulative brain injury. The design of the boxing glove has been significantly altered to reduce impact. In both amateur and professional boxing, the referee, trainer and doctor will stop a fight earlier than used to occur. In amateur boxing outside the UK, many competitions now insist on the participants wearing protective headgear, but these have not been subjected to the same detailed scrutiny to check their efficacy

159
Chapter 10
The doctor's
contribution
towards safety in
sport

160

Chapter 10
The doctor's
contribution
towards safety in
sport

as has been applied to the skull-cap worn by jockeys and the helmets worn in American football or ice-hockey ·

Ice-hockey

Ice-hockey is a fast, exciting sport, inevitably involving contact through collision. Violence has all too readily been accepted, if not actively encouraged, to draw in the crowds. This violence has been associated with well-documented cases of catastrophic injury, particularly in North America, and this has led to increasing medical concern as to the standard of supervision of the sport and the enforcement of the rules under which it should be played. Ongoing studies continue into the incidence of serious injury in ice-hockey and there is great concern associated with the number of players suffering quadriplegia following a crash into the boards at the side of the rink, after they have been pushed or 'checked' from behind.

International sport

International travel in sport and the consequent problems of alteration in the participant's biorhythm due to jet lag, acclimatisation and changes in altitude are other areas in which the interested doctor can be involved in the prevention of injuries or illness. Detailed studies in this field have been undertaken, particularly with regard to athletics and cycling. These studies have shown that even the fittest athletes must allow one day's recovery for every three- to four-hour adjustment in their 'time clock', whether they are travelling east or west from their normal time-zone environment. Additional stresses will be placed on athletes if they ascend to an altitude of over 1000 m, or if there is a significant change in either the temperature or the humidity. A doctor helping prepare athletes for a significant competition on the other side of the world or in another environment will be involved in detailed planning with the athlete and his or her coach, with regard to modification of the athlete's training programme, diet, salt and water intake during the crucial acclimatisation period, as well as ensuring that the athlete rapidly returns to a normal pattern of sleeping and waking. Failure to undertake this planning inevitably results in overuse injuries, principally to muscles and tendons, an increased vulnerability to direct injury as a result of fatigue, and the danger of 'metabolic collapse'.

Hill-walking

The report prepared by the Medical Adviser to the Scottish Mountain Rescue Committee on the nature of causes of injuries sustained in 190 Scottish mountain accidents is a prime example of what can be achieved as a result of informed analysis of appropriate injuries. This report highlights a series of risk factors among which it states that the commonest cause of injury while hill-walking in Scotland is a simple slip or stumble and that there is a need for increased awareness among the public of the risks that they take. Avalanches are a major cause of winter mountain accidents in Scotland and widespread education initiatives have been taken to draw attention to the frequency, causes and risks of avalanches in Scotland throughout the winter. An avalanche, in conjunction with the failure to carry and to be competent in the use of crampons or ice-axes, invariably leads to a fatal accident.

161
*Chapter 10
The doctor's
contribution
towards safety in
sport*

Conclusion

Many governing bodies in sport have yet to develop appropriate medical advisory services. Such a service will have various administrative and organisational responsibilities but one of the most worthwhile contributions that the medical profession can make to sport is to undertake relevant research into the incidence of injury and illness associated with that sport, with a view to identifying risk factors that result in injury that can readily be eliminated from the sport in question without altering the character of that sport. Sport for all need not necessarily mean minor injuries for many, moderate injuries for some, permanent disability for a few and the occasional death, if the sports legislators have the relevant risk factors drawn to their attention by informed and committed doctors working with them.

References

McGregor A. R. (1988) The nature and cause of injuries sustained in 190 Scottish mountain accidents. *Scottish Sports Council Research Digest*, No. 1.
Schneider *et al.* (1985) *Sports Injuries: Mechanisms, Prevention and Treatment*, eds Schneider *et al.* Baltimore: Williams & Watkins.

11 Fatalities associated with sport

BERNARD KNIGHT

'Death is the great leveller'
J. Kelly, Scottish proverb

Incidence of fatalities

No reliable overall mortality statistics are available for sporting activities. Apart from the inherent errors in all mortality figures, due to inaccurate certification, many sport-associated deaths are not identifiable as such in official statistics. For example, 'natural' deaths precipitated by exertion are usually registered solely under the disease process. Deaths of spectators may not be categorised under a sport index — and many deaths directly attributable to sporting activity may not be identifiable from the raw statistical material.

Where legal inquiries are made, primarily coroner's inquests in England, Wales and Ireland, a study of the annual returns provides reliable information — but, where the cause of death is recorded as 'natural causes', no such inquest is held.*

Though overall statistics are unsatisfactory, some idea of the relative risks to life of the various sports may be gained from figures attributed to certain categories, and these will be mentioned later under the appropriate headings. In general, the greatest single cause of mortality associated with sporting activities is undoubtedly pre-existing natural disease exacerbated by exertion. This far exceeds trauma and other causes directly attributable to the performance of sport.

*Certification of death should be made by the 'ordinary medical attendant' of the patients, in cases where the death is not reported to the coroner. For further details, see p. 163.

The legal aspects of sporting fatalities

Before discussing the actual causes of death in various sports, the legal consequences must be surveyed. There are a number of aspects which may affect the doctor, whether he or she is a team medical officer, the medical attendant of an individual competitor or merely a doctor who only becomes involved when some tragedy occurs.

Death certification

If the death undoubtedly appears due to natural disease, then certification will depend upon the particular circumstances. If the deceased's own medical attendant is called, he or she may — and indeed may be obliged to — provide a medical certification of the cause of death if it is known that the patient suffered from some potentially fatal disease and he or she had attended the deceased at some time in the two weeks before death. If the doctor considers that the circumstances are quite consistent with death from the pre-existing disease, then certification must proceed as in any other natural death, irrespective of the sporting connection. It is debatable whether or not a team doctor can be considered to be 'the medical attendant', if the victim has another regular doctor such as a home general practitioner. Before any doctor can sign a death certificate, acceptable to the registrar of births and deaths, he or she must have seen the deceased in a professional capacity during the 14 days immediately preceding the death, which also means that he or she must be fully aware of the medical history, if any.

Probably, if a person dies whilst taking part in an event taking place near home, his/her own GP should sign the certificate if he or she saw the deceased during the past fortnight, provided that the death is not to be reported to the coroner. If death occurs at some sporting event away from home, then it will depend on the attitude of the local coroner as to whether he or she would consider the team medical officer to be 'the medical attendant'. In many (probably most) cases, the coroner would require the death to be formally reported to him or her, so that an autopsy could be conducted. If death occurs abroad, then the local regulations will apply, and these will vary from country to country.

Reporting to the coroner

Even where death seems due to natural causes, if it is sudden and unexpected, most will need to be reported to the coroner, in England, Wales, Ulster and the Irish Republic. In Scotland, the Procurator-fiscal is the corresponding law officer.

Only if the deceased had a well-diagnosed disease which was recognised as lethal — and the doctor had attended him/her professionally during the past 14 days and the circumstances of the death seem consistent with the diagnosis — can a coroner's inquiry be avoided. In most cases associated with sport, this would hardly apply, as someone with such recently diagnosed and treated serious disease is unlikely to be indulging in strenuous activity — although of course it does happen.

Reporting a death to the coroner is usually carried out by the police where trauma or other accident has occurred. If natural disease is suspected, but the doctor cannot provide a valid certificate, either because of the 14-day rule or because it is felt that the sporting activity has had a contributory effect, he or she may well telephone the coroner, usually via the coroner's officer or other policemen.*

In jurisdictions other than Britain, the local regulations will apply. In the USA, some states have a coroner system, but many

* In cases of doubt it is always wiser for the doctor concerned to discuss the case with the coroner via the coroner's officer. The doctor may wish to seek advice initially from his protection organisation.

have a Medical Examiner Office, where the forensic pathologist is also the equivalent of the coroner, combining the medical and circumstantial investigation.

In many parts of the Commonwealth, the British coroner system remains a legacy of empire, but in most of Europe, the police and a judge assume the central role in the investigation of sudden, un-expected or traumatic deaths.

Whatever the system, witnesses will be required to give state-ments of their knowledge of the events surrounding the death and one of the prime witnesses will be the doctor. He or she will have to relate the medical knowledge of the deceased, including the clinical history and the mode of death, etc.

Medical confidentiality is not usually a consideration in a coroner's inquiry, as all witnesses can be obliged by subpoena to attend an inquest and be compelled to divulge any information to which they are privy, on pain of penalties for contempt of court.

In all cases of traumatic or unnatural death, an inquest will be held, almost inevitably after an autopsy. Unless a doctor has been able to issue a death certificate in the cases of natural death, these will also be reported to the coroner and an autopsy performed. If the latter reveals that death was due to natural disease, the coroner will dispose of the case and issue a certificate, in most cases without an inquest. However, some natural deaths associated with sport will still go to a public inquest, either because the law statutorily re-quires this or because the coroner's discretionary powers persuade him or her to hold an inquest.

For example, a man who suddenly drops dead playing squash and whose autopsy reveals a recent myocardial infarct is unlikely to be the subject of an inquest. However, the death of the same man whose infarct causes him to crash his competition glider must go to an inquest — and an inquest with jury — as this is statutorily classed as an aviation fatality. Yet again, if the same man died during the same squash game, with the same infarct, but his wife complained that the doctor was negligent in not diagnosing his coronary disease the previous month, then the coroner may well exercise his or her discretion in holding an inquest to clarify the situation.*

When a death is reported to the coroner, whether or not an inquest is held, the doctor has no further part to play other than providing a statement and probably appearing as a witness. The

---

*At such an inquest the family of the deceased may well be represented by solicitors and/or barristers. Such 'high-profile' proceedings may well indicate the subsequent intention of civil proceedings directed against the medical attendant(s) of the deceased. If the doctor finds himself unexpectedly under attack at an inquest, it is advisable to request an adjournment to permit the doctor to seek legal advice and/or representation.

doctor does not sign a death certificate or a cremation certificate, as these are provided by the coroner.

Civil liability

Where one person brings a legal action for damages against another, the suit is a civil matter as opposed to criminal proceedings, in which one party is the State, acting in the name of the sovereign.

In sport it has been accepted for centuries that someone who voluntarily participates does so under the mutual understanding that he or she accepts any risk arising from that sport, including the actions of other players who are participating in the game. A rock-climber who falls from a cliff-face cannot sue the owner of the mountain; nor can a boxer who suffers a subdural haematoma sue his opponent. This concept is embodied in the maxim *volenti non fit injuria*.

Of course, injuries or death sustained during a sporting activity only come under this dictum if they were suffered during the normal course of the sport. If a rugby player has some ribs broken in a legitimate tackle, he cannot sue the other player — but, if the other player breaks his jaw with a deliberate punch, this would be grounds for an action in tort — and perhaps also for a criminal prosecution (see pp. 51–63).

This long-standing 'gentlemen's agreement' has gained the force of law over the years, it being accepted that every sports man or woman carries his or her own risks. However, this has been challenged in recent years by an increasing number of cases in which injury or death has been blamed on the actions of others. The injured party or the personal representatives of a dead player may sue another player for negligence or assault, relying mainly on a departure from the accepted rules and conduct of the game, to avoid the *volenti non fit injuria* concept, for the basis of their case.

Of course, civil actions may also be brought against the manufacturers of allegedly faulty equipment which has led to mishaps — the snapping of a weak wire on a hang-glider or a badly designed face-mask on an American footballer may lead to an action in contract or tort against the manufacturer, or an action under any relevant product liability legislation.

In all these matters, the doctor may become involved in giving an opinion on the mode of causation of the injury or death or in describing his or her part in attempted resuscitation and treatment. The doctor may alternatively be the party sued, if it is alleged, for example, that he or she:

1 allowed an unfit player to go on the field or participate in some hazardous activity such as diving or climbing, etc.;

2 was negligent in diagnosis, treatment or resuscitatory measures after the mishap occurred.

The fact that a team or club doctor is usually an unpaid volunteer makes no difference to his duty of professional care to a patient. The three essentials of negligence — medical or otherwise — are that:

1 the defendant (doctor) has a duty of care to the plaintiff (patient), and

2 there is a breach of that duty, by an act either of commission or of omission, and

3 the patient suffered damage as a result — in this context, death. Though the deceased patient is obviously unable to take legal action him or herself, the personal representative of the deceased may sue, the bulk of the potential damages being recompense for lost earning capacity for benefit of dependent relatives.[*]

Criminal proceedings

Until very recently, it was virtually unheard of for criminal proceedings to arise from injuries in sport, as the spirit of the *volenti non fit injuria* principle made it even less likely that the State would interest itself in such a matter. Though not involving deaths, several recent events of a somewhat shameful nature on the rugby field have ended in criminal prosecutions and convictions (see pp. 14–26). This unhappy development is perhaps symptomatic of the erosion of the sporting ethos consequent upon the increasing pressure to win, rather than the rather more old-fashioned acceptance of 'taking part' as the important feature of sport.

Violently frayed tempers lead to personal combat on the field and the cases referred to criminal proceedings have included the partial biting off of an ear and other injuries sustained in a common assault. The only relevance to the doctor involved in these types of cases would be the probability of his being called either as a witness as to fact from seeing what happened or, more likely, as a professional witness to describe the original appearance of the injuries.

Natural disease and sporting deaths

The great majority of sport-associated fatalities are due to pre-existing natural disease, rather than trauma and other unnatural processes. The deaths are usually sudden and unexpected, as people with overtly dangerous symptoms are unlikely to indulge in strenuous sporting pastimes.

---

[*] This is because sport as a leisure activity is predominantly a pastime of young, fit, employed individuals. Loss of earnings — usually calculated as the annual sum lost (the multiplicand) multiplied by the remaining life expectancy in years (the multiplier) — is often a large sum of money, for which the doctor may be liable if negligence and causation are proven.

As with most sudden unexpected deaths, the prime cause lies in the cardiovascular system, even if the blood vessels responsible lie not necessarily in the thorax, but in the cranium or abdomen.

Coronary atherosclerosis

This is not exactly synonymous with 'ischaemic heart disease' because other cardiac diseases, such as hypertension, aortic valve disease and some congenital abnomalies, also cause myocardial ischaemia. Nor is it equivalent to 'coronary thrombosis' or 'myocardial infarction', both of which, where no autopsy has been performed, are over-diagnosed as causes of sudden death. In fact, the mode of coronary death likely to be associated with strenuous sporting activity is not that of a myocardial infarct, which is usually a sequel to thrombus formation or an atheromatous stenosis.

The coroner's pathologist sees a different population of coronary victims than does the hospital physician, and is forced to assume that sudden, unexpected death is more often due to an arrythmia, such as ventricular fibrillation, producing cardiac arrest. People who die from established coronary thrombi and infarcts are more likely to die in front of their television sets than on a jogging circuit, though of course it cannot be denied that some such deaths are precipitated by exercise when morphological myocardial damage already exists.

The effect of catecholamines, noradrenaline, etc., is probably relevant to sudden death in sport, because adrenal activity from emotion, excitement and competitive exertion is more likely to induce ventricular arrythmias in susceptible individuals. Recent observations on the use of injected catecholamines in attempted resuscitation have shown that myocardial fibres can be rapidly damaged, with the formation of fragmented myofibrils with contraction bands. The cardiac arrythmias seen in solvent abuse have been shown to be due to these substances sensitising the myocardium to noradrenaline.

It is beyond the scope of this text to describe the symptomatology and pathology of coronary artery disease, but suffice to say, that numerically, it forms the greater part of sport-associated sudden deaths.

Within this group, the doctor must be alert for the victim of familial hypercholesterolaemia because of the need for subsequent diagnosis and prophylactic measures amongst the surviving family. This diagnosis will rest on autopsy findings and all young persons dying of coronary atheroma below the age of 35 should have post-mortem cholesterol levels measured. It is one of the few biochemical analyses which give reliable results *post mortem* and is an example of the community health benefits that can flow from coroner's pathology.

Other cardiac conditions

In older age-groups, hypertensive heart disease and calcific aortic stenosis are relatively common causes of sudden unexpected death. In younger persons, the whole range of cardiomyopathies may be encountered, including asymmetric septal hypertrophy or hypertrophic obstructive cardiomyopathy (HOCM). These are usually unsuspected and therefore undiagnosed in people who are characteristically asymptomatic and thus well enough to participate in active sports.

Some years ago, 'isolated, Fiedler's or Saphir's myocarditis' was a favourite diagnosis for sudden deaths in young subjects, being based on the histological detection of foci of chronic inflammatory cells in the myocardium. Many of the diagnoses were based on insufficient evidence and some published surveys of traffic fatalities have shown that similar patchy cellular infiltrates are present in control populations.

Congenital cardiac lesions are occasionally found in sport-associated deaths, especially atrial septal defects, patent ductus arteriosus, coarctation of the aorta and various valve defects. Death may occur even when these conditions are already diagnosed: the risk of acute cardiac failure can be underestimated. Other cases are found for the first time at autopsy.

Obscure cardiac deaths

Every coroner's pathologist sees a few deaths each year in which the most exhaustive investigation fails to reveal the cause of death. Even excluding the most common group of this type, namely the so-called 'cot deaths' in infants, most of the obscure cases are in young people, both teenagers and young adults. This section of the population will obviously contain some sport-related deaths simply because the age range coincides. One cannot, however, deduce any causal relationship with sport in these fatalities.

It is probable that these obscure deaths occur also in older subjects, but there is often an overlay of chronic degenerative cardiovascular disease, notably coronary atheroma, which provides an acceptable and convenient, if not always wholly convincing, reason for the death.

These deaths of occult cause may occur on or off the sports arena. In some instances, a footballer or runner may literally drop dead on the field, obviously the victim of a cardiac arrest. Due to the lack of any premonitory symptoms, there is no opportunity to determine whether some arrythymia preceded the collapse. In other cases, the death may occur some time after the actual sporting exertion and here it is extremely questionable as to whether the fatality can be linked in any way with the activity. For example, the author dealt with the death of a previously fit young man of 21, who played a Saturday afternoon game of club rugby. He celebrated in moderation that evening, then awoke during the night with non-specific complaints of feeling unwell — then promptly died. A full autopsy with histology, virology, toxicology and microbiology failed to reveal the slightest abnormality and the death had to be recorded as 'unascertained'.

Lesions of large arteries

Rupture of an aortic aneurysm is a common cause of sudden, un-expected death in the general population but again is relatively unlikely to be seen very often in active participants of the more strenuous types of sports, because these lesions are more common in advancing age. However, many men in their fifties and sixties may be at risk whilst jogging, playing squash or taking part in strenuous exercise, especially if it is unaccustomed.

The most common type of aortic aneurysm occurs as a result of an atheromatous degeneration. This is most commonly found in the abdominal segment of the vessel, though it can occur in its thoracic course.

Less often, a dissection of an aorta suffering from medionecrosis may occur, although the event is precipitated by a tear through an atheromatous plaque on the inner surface. Dissecting aneurysms are usually in the thoracic aorta, though they may rapidly spread upwards and downwards, often leading to aortic incompetence and cardiac tamponade if the upper extension enters the pericardial sac.

Rarely, a young person may be struck with a dissecting aneurysm as part of a Marfan-type syndrome.

Cerebral aneurysms — subarachnoid haemorrhage

One of the major causes of sudden disability and death in young and middle-aged adults is subarachnoid bleeding, almost always from a ruptured berry aneurysm on the circle of Willis.

This affects both sexes and, because of the relative immunity of younger women from fatal coronary disease, it is one of the first causes to consider in the sudden unexpected death of a woman under the age of 45 — the other causes being pulmonary embolism and complications of pregnancy.

The pathology is well known and needs no further elaboration here. The aneurysms are sometimes called 'congenital', but this description is not accurate, as they develop as age progresses. The weakness in the arterial wall, however, is congenital, probably due to fenestration in the elastic laminae at the site of atrophied foetal vessels.

In a small proportion of 'spontaneous' subarachnoid haemorrhage (i.e. known to be unassociated with trauma), no aneurysm is detected at autopsy, but this is in part due to the difficulties of identifying a small lesion after rupture. About 15% of non-traumatic subarachnoid haemorrhages are not associated with a discoverable aneurysm.

The precipitating factors in the rupture of a cerebral aneurysm are only partly understood. A rise in blood-pressure is undoubtedly a potent factor and, in view of the number of dramatic collapses and some deaths that have occurred on the sports field, it seems likely that strenuous physical exertion must be related. Whether it is a rise in systolic and diastolic blood-pressure or a marked increase in heart rate and cardiac output is not known.

Obviously excitement and emotion, with their adrenal response, are as potent as muscular exertion. Of course, as with coronary and other cardiovascular disease, a berry aneurysm can rupture at rest, but proof that intense and perhaps unaccustomed exercise is a factor is shown by the not uncommon history of collapse and sometimes death during sexual intercourse.

There is a controversy in the forensic world about the role of alcohol in the rupture of a berry aneurysm. It is claimed, unconvincingly, that alcohol both increases the blood-pressure and dilates the cerebral vessels: in fact, alcohol widens the pulse pressure somewhat, but may actually lower the diastolic pressure. As for dilating cerebral vessels, the completely fibrotic sac of a cerebral aneurysm is quite incapable of muscular vasodilatation.

More pertinent than alcohol in relation to sports fatalities is the role of trauma in ruptured cerebral aneurysms. It is hard to deny that an expanded, thin-walled aneurysmal sac is vulnerable to the physical trauma that accompanies many sports, especially boxing and rugby football. Only a few years ago, a rugby player of international renown was struck down during a match with a ruptured 'berry' aneurysm, thankfully surviving long enough to undergo successful neurosurgery. It may be noteworthy, however, that the haemorrhage which occurred was unassociated with head trauma immediately prior to the player's collapse on the field of play.

In the criminal sphere, which might have future relevance to sporting injuries, it has been a matter of considerable controversy as to whether the perpetrator of an assault which was followed by a fatal rupture of a cerebral aneurysm could be charged with homicide. In England (as opposed to Scotland or the Continent), it was formerly held that there was reasonable doubt about the causative connection between a ruptured berry aneurysm and head trauma, but several cases in recent years have tended to strengthen the association between the two.

The issue of causation, in berry aneurysm, is of relevance in the sporting context, when it has to be decided, either by a coroner, a court or some internal sporting inquiry, whether the fatality was indeed a consequence of a head injury. Because of the undoubted association with exertion and emotion, which may be impossible to separate in time from the actual injury, it may be difficult indeed to decide on causation.

Another important association with subarachnoid haemorrhage is trauma to the side of the neck. Unrecognised until a few years ago, this probably accounted for some of the cases of 'spontaneous' subarachnoid bleeding where no aneurysm was found. The pathologist in a proportion of these occult cases probably missed deep bruising in the neck muscles behind and below the ear, as this is an area which is not usually dissected by the pathologist unless there are specific indications. The lesion in these catastrophes is a tear in a vertebral artery, which allows blood to track into the cranial cavity at the level of the foramen magnum. Most of the early published cases had a fracture of the transverse process of the atlas vertebra, but later it was shown that such a fracture is not necessary for the damage to the vertebral artery either in the osseous tunnel or where it perforates the dura. The injury to the neck need not be severe — it seems to be the specificity of the target area that is important, causing acute lateral flexion and rotation of the head on the upper cervical vertebrae, with possibly stretching of the atlanto-occipital membrane. The lesion is seen quite often in criminal assaults and, although no case has been reported in the forensic literature as having occurred in a sporting context, it is likely that some past subarachnoid haemorrhages have been misdiagnosed, where the relatively mild injury to the neck has been unrecorded.

Other natural causes

Though persons with chronic diseases in general have to either avoid or reduce their participation in sporting activities, there has been a marked trend recently for people with all kinds and degrees of disability to involve themselves in many types of sport. Here the doctor has a vital role in tailoring their activities to their capabilities and in detecting early signs of their exceeding their threshold of safety.

However, even with the most vigilant monitoring, sudden deterioration, even to the point of death, may occur in a variety of natural diseases. For example, sudden death may supervene, in a sporting context as well as elsewhere, in patients with bronchial asthma or epilepsy. An asthmatic may die quite unexpectedly, even if he or she is not in status asthmaticus or perhaps not even suffering an attack. Once again, the sensitisation of the myocardium by adrenergic bronchodilators must always be suspect as a cause of sudden arrythmia and arrest — a syndrome which caused many deaths some 20 years ago, until intense medical publicity reduced the usage of adrenergic drugs in the treatment of asthma. Even where such toxic effects can be excluded, asthma can still lead to unexpected death, and the same applies to epilepsy, where a sudden fatality may be unassociated with status epilepticus or even a solitary fit.

In summary, many types of natural disease may cause death, either in the infinite variety of situations of daily life or in the sporting context. It may be impossible to distinguish these, as it may be sheer chance that a probably inevitable death happened to occur whilst the victim was indulging in some sporting activity.

The many spectators who die of cardiovascular disease and those who die whilst performing some non-strenuous pastime would perhaps have died elsewhere at the same time. However, the wrestler who dies of acute cardiac insufficiency during a bout or the weight-lifter who ruptures an aneurysm whilst in competition almost certainly has had his fatal event precipitated by exertion.

Intermediate between these is the situation where, though the physical stress is minimal, there is an element of excitement and emotion which may mediate itself through the adrenal response to trigger the fatal episode. In determining the cause and effect, which may well have legal repercussions of greater or lesser degree, the facts of each tragedy must be assessed in an individual way.

Further reading

Cameron J. M. & Mant A. K. (1972) Fatal subarachnoid haemorrhage associated with cervical trauma. *Medicine, Science and Law* **12**, 66–70.

Coast G. C. & Gee D. J. (1984) Traumatic subarachnoid haemorrhage — an alternative source. *Journal of Clinical Pathology* **37**, 1245.

Karch S. B. (1987) Resuscitation induced myocardial necrosis, catecholamines and defibrillation. *American Journal of Forensic Medicine and Pathology* **8**, 3–8.

Simonsen J. (1988) Massive subarachnoid haemorrhage: report of six cases and a review of the literature. *American Journal of Forensic Medicine and Pathology* **9**, 23–31.

Athletes at an overseas venue: the role of the team doctor 12

M. BOTTOMLEY

'''"What matters it how far we go"
his scaly friend replied,
"there is another shore you know
upon the other side.
The further off from England,
the nearer is to France.
Then turn not pale beloved snail
but come and join the dance"''
From *Alice in Wonderland* by Lewis Caroll

It is a great privilege to be asked to be a team doctor whether it be for the local rugby club or an Olympic team. As part of an international team one is also entrusted with a considerable responsibility, not only to keep the athletes going, but also to protect them against long-term harm that could, amongst other considerations, involve large sums of money in terms of potential earnings and sponsor's investment.[*]

[*] The doctor's responsibility is, however, primarily towards the individual team member as his 'patient'.

Sports Medicine is a speciality. There are now two Diploma examinations in the subject, that of the London Hospital being preceded by an academic year of full-time study, whilst the Diploma of the Society of Apothecaries can be taken following one of several part-time courses. Other Diploma examinations and courses are in the planning stage. Few official team Medical Officers are qualified in this way. Most have their grounding in the British Association of Sport and Medicine's one week residential introductory and advanced courses.[*] This may be topped up by attending such lectures and short courses as may crop up locally, together with reading articles and the few available textbooks. It is important to be interested in the problems peculiar to sport and to have a very real sympathy with the aims of the athlete. School or university doctors often develop an interest as an inevitable part of their job; others may have enjoyed success in sport themselves and have a particular empathy with sporting patients.

There is no career structure in sports medicine. For most it is a 'hobby' which just about pays for itself through sports injury clinics

[*] Further details about these courses can be obtained from the Education Officer, British Association of Sport and Medicine, c/o the London Sports Medicine Institute, St Bartholomew's Hospital, Charterhouse Square, London EC1M 6BQ.

173

174

Chapter 12
Athletes at an
overseas venue:
the role of the
team doctor

or, rarely, through a retainer paid by a club. Team doctors are not paid. Whilst it is true that reasonable expenses are claimable and all fares and accommodation are provided, most team doctors find that, in the long run, they are out of pocket. Absence from professional practice for prolonged periods of time during major championships is an inevitable demand which will draw heavily on holiday entitlement. Colleagues' co-operation to provide cover is an essential requirement. Drugs and treatments can be claimed as expenses, but more often than not it is the practice drug cupboard or the hospital that replenishes the team doctor's bag.

The team doctor, having been invited by the club or governing body of the sport in question, is acting as an agent of that club or body. There is no formal contract. The British Amateur Athletic Board, to which the author is a medical officer, relies largely on the goodwill of its medical officers, who are regarded as team officials. As such, they are covered by insurance for both personal ill health and for loss of personal property whilst abroad.

Athletes are very mobile people in many senses of the word, often competing and training all over Europe, if not the world. They are therefore exposed to a wide variety of medical opinion and will tend to seek out doctors whom they perceive as sympathetic to their needs, often being prepared to travel considerable distances. At every competition the organisers will have provided local medical and physiotherapy cover; at major competitions this may be supplemented by medical or paramedical services provided by equipment firms. Since the official team doctor is taken only on international representative trips and since there is no central system of record keeping, the medical care of athletes is likely to be haphazard and fragmentary.

The team doctor's role

The team doctor's job begins well before a trip. Although some of the team may be seasoned travellers there may well be others who are going abroad for the first time. Some kind of preparatory advice is always useful, both to remind the experienced and to inform the innocent.

The extent of the advice depends very much on the venue, but if travelling outside Europe recommendations on preparatory inoculations,* comfortable aircraft travel and minimising the effects of jet lag should be offered. Some advice on food hygiene may be appropriate as well as any special risks there may be in the area,

---

*Advice on inoculations is published regularly in various medical newspapers, notably *Pulse*, and in the DH booklets SA40 and SA41. Further information is in the book *Traveller's Health* by Richard Dawood, published by Oxford University Press. Specific advice on malaria requirements is obtainable from: 071–637 7921 (taped message, 24-hour service) or 071–637 0248 (Egypt, Morocco and Turkey only).

e.g. rabies. Many athletes like to jog as part of their preparation and runners seem to have a magnetic attraction for dogs.

Weather and insect pests may be important. The athlete will probably have been briefed by his coach about climate, heat and humidity, but the doctor should be prepared to deal with any problems that may arise. If conditions are anticipated to be extreme it is hoped that the athlete has a chance to acclimatise.

A reminder about AIDS is not inappropriate in a situation where healthy young men and women from all parts of the world come together in an atmosphere of instant camaraderie (see Chapter 8).

Travelling as part of a large group will present logistic and organisational problems. The team doctor is always appreciated that bit more if he or she is willing to help. Such things as sorting out tickets, labelling luggage and negotiating with airline staff as to how the vaulters' poles can be handled or whether a javelin constitutes an offensive weapon are an inevitable part of any journey.

You may prefer to keep your medical bag as hand luggage or it may go into the hold. However, it is always as well to have some simple remedies to hand. The travel-sick may not have their favourite treatment, or the dysmenorrhoeic their pain-killer. Travel breeds headache and sleeplessness. Some paracetamol and a short-acting mild sedative* are therefore useful. It is important to ensure that your medical kit is available at times when it is required. You do tend to feel a bit inadequate if you have to confess that all your medical kit is locked away in the bowels of the aircraft.

Athletes are notoriously conservative about their diet and many will reject the very different foods that they are offered in, say, eastern Europe or Japan. Team doctors may well find that they are having to negotiate to try and provide more familiar foods and may even need to forage the local supermarket for supplies.

The team doctor is there to be available. It may at times seem that athletes are unreasonably demanding in their needs. If they want treatment, for whatever reason, they want it then and there so that their preparation schedule is not interrupted. In the opinion of the author, a competitor who has spent months or years training for an event does have a right to unlimited access to the team medical officer for treatment. It is important, therefore, that the team knows where you are at all times.

It is important also to remain 'one of the team' and thus it is essential not to appear aloof whilst at the same time maintaining professional detachment.

Accommodation overseas varies considerably. For the most part teams stay in good-quality hotels, which, at the more important events, may be designated as the competition village. For events such as the Olympics the accommodation may be purpose-built and used subsequently as housing stock for the host city.

It is unusual to have a separate treatment room where you are

*Opinions vary, but the author finds that temazepam is satisfactory; it is available as a 10 mg capsule. Loprazolam, lormetazepam and triazolam are similarly acting drugs.

176

*Chapter 12
Athletes at an
overseas venue:
the role of the
team doctor*

staying; neither is any equipment supplied. Your bed, or even, occasionally, the vanitory unit top, provides an examination or treatment couch. At major international events there may well be a medical centre in the village, which is usually staffed by the host country.

The organising committee will have made some provisions for medical care at the track, but it can be very variable, ranging from a couch in the corner of the dressing-room to a fully manned medical centre. Apart from the highly prestigious events, it is unusual to have any prior information as to what is available, so that a preliminary inspection of the arena is worth while. Even then it is unlikely that any responsible official will be available for advice so that the medical officer may have to wait until the technical meeting held by officials before the event to find out what medical facilities there are.

Ideally the organisers should have provided a track clearance team to transfer an injured athlete to the medical centre. An ambulance should also be available for evacuation to hospital where appropriate. The medical officer should know where the nearest hospital is and the facilities that they offer. In Japan, for instance, there can be difficulty in obtaining treatment at certain hospitals as a foreigner; it is necessary for the medical officer to be aware of the local rules. It is therefore important also to know where in the stadium the nearest phone is and how to use it, and to have some local currency handy.

At the best of times consultations will be relatively informal — in the hotel bedroom or a medical room at the stadium. Frequently, however, they can take place at the track side, in the bar or on the coach. Whilst it is generally better if privacy can be provided, one often finds in the gregarious atmosphere of a team that the patients are quite happy to be seen and treated in the midst of a crowd. This cannot always be taken for granted, however, and an alert eye must be kept open for those who really do prefer some privacy.

Athletes in general are a healthy group of people, but they are just as liable to minor illness as anyone else, and, indeed, may be more at risk than normally through being away from their normal environment. Certain more chronic diseases are not incompatible with sport at the highest level and athletes may be asthmatic, diabetic or even epileptic.

The health problems are mainly those familiar to any GP and the medical bag should reflect this. One important consideration is, however, that international athletes are subject to strict rules limiting the treatments they may have. The logic of these rules is not always immediately obvious but nevertheless the team medical officer should be totally familiar with the list of banned substances laid down by the sports governing body. In terms of day-to-day treatment, that principally means ephedrine and its derivatives, together with codeine and caffeine, all present in many cold cures and pain-killers. Since these are sold widely over the counter the team doctor should insist that the athletes declare any treatments that they are having or have recently had.

There are, of course, problems related directly to sport. Injuries are common, but most of these are of a minor nature and affect soft tissues, often not amounting to more than localised stiffness. Whilst these injuries would pass unnoticed in the average individual, to an athlete performing at maximum physical effort they represent a source of serious anxiety or may even cause actual inhibition of function.

The physiotherapist is often the hardest-worked member of the team but simple massage should be well within the capabilities of the team doctor and it allows the physiotherapist to get on with more specialised treatments. The 'hands-on' experience is useful in many ways. Apart from the obvious relief to the athlete, it gives the doctor a real appreciation of what the athlete means when he describes a tight spot in a muscle. Often one can feel it relax as treatment is applied. It also helps in getting to know the athlete. The physiotherapy room often seems to be a social centre and chatting to the patients during treatment helps them to relax. A knowledge of some simple strapping techniques can also be useful.

Treatment is not necessarily aimed at helping the athlete to continue. There are certain situations where continued competiton will make matters worse. It is something that ought to be discussed with the athlete and perhaps also with the coach and team manager. The ultimate choice has to be that of the athlete, but the doctor should never be persuaded into treatment that allows the athlete to compete at the risk of worsening his or her condition. My own feeling is that local anaesthetics and local steroid injections are, as a general rule, best left at home, particularly as far as short trips are concerned.

The treatment that is given for anything other than minor problems may be looked on as 'first aid'. The aims of treatment are to prevent the condition getting worse and to establish a solid base for rehabilitation. Whilst in general terms rehabilitation is going to be along predictable lines, it is not fair on your colleagues who are going to do most of the work in getting the athlete better to commit them too specifically to a particular treatment.

Keeping comprehensive records is not easy. It is important, though, that you keep a record of your own management. This should include every patient that you see, which may include athletes of other countries who seek your help, since not all teams bring their own doctor. No standard form of record is available and it is probably easier to keep a diary or daybook from which information can be transferred to a more formal file if you wish. There are signs that, in the increasingly professional world of sport, medico-

177
Chapter 12
Athletes at an
overseas venue:
the role of the
team doctor

178

*Chapter 12
Athletes at an
overseas venue:
the role of the
team doctor*

legal problems are cropping up and, without a record of your management, your position might be difficult to defend.*

One solution that has been suggested to the vexed problem of keeping a comprehensive record is that athletes are given their own case notes which they produce every time they are treated. Unless each doctor or physiotherapist keeps a duplicate of his or her own notes that would create enormous difficulties in the event of any dispute over treatment. A central record, held by the governing body, with appropriate notes being carried to a meeting and returned by a responsible official would be more satisfactory, but would involve considerable administrative costs.

The professional relationship that exists between the team doctor and the athletes is akin to that of a factory medical officer* and its employees, although, when abroad, the function is extended since the doctor also has to act as the 'GP'. One of the problems in dealing with athletes is that doctors in general have a poor reputation in the treatment of sports-related problems. Many colleagues still take the view that they are self-limiting disorders that will eventually heal if they are not further provoked. Not only is this untrue but totally neglects the athlete's need for a speedy and total recovery.

Referral of an injured athlete after a competition therefore raises a number of ethical problems. Advice to return to his or her own GP may well be rejected and ignored. If specialist help is necessary the GP may not know of an appropriate opinion. Physiotherapy is a vital ingredient in rehabilitation but by no means every physiotherapist is equipped to deal with the particular problems arising from sport.

The world of sports medicine is relatively small and those who work in it are generally known to each other and to the athletes. It is therefore likely that many athletes will refer themselves to an appropriate opinion, with or without the collusion of the team doctor, and the GP may well be bypassed. One of the great strengths of our system of medical care is that the GP remains at the heart of management and that specialists on the whole insist on GP referral whether it be through the NHS or privately. It is a great pity that the treatment of athletes undermines this principle but until sports medicine achieves a legitimate status this untidy situation is likely to persist.

The team doctor's bag is as idiosyncratic as general practice. In addition to emergency treatments for conditions like asthma, diabetes, severe pain or anaphylaxis it is useful to be able to deal with

---

*This being the case, the team doctor ought, in theory at least, to correspond with the athlete's own GP on returning home, notifying any treatment given, etc.

---

*The Medical Protection Society provides legal advice and the opportunity to apply for indemnity against professional negligence for doctors all parts of the world except USA and Canada. When visiting North American or Canada, therefore, it would be prudent to establish with the organisers beforehand the extent of the legal cover which they would be prepared to provide.

179

Chapter 12
Athletes at an
overseas venue:
the role of the
team doctor

some of the simpler problems. The common cold, hay fever, indigestion, gastroenteritis, ear infections, cuts, blisters and bruises are all as common in athletes as in any other section of the population. In some countries insect bites can be a major problem, both from the irritation they cause and because of the risk of infection, so that some repellent cream and/or sprays may be helpful. If one sees simple physiotherapy as part of one's role, an assortment of strappings and various 'rubs' will also be useful.

The bag may well contain certain controlled drugs, such as pethidine. A Home Office licence, valid for the appropriate period, should be obtained before taking such drugs abroad in order to satisfy HM Customs, and clearance should be obtained in advance from the embassies of the countries to be visited. In practice customs officials tend to be tolerant towards teams and team doctors, which obviously implies a trust, and that should not be abused. Host countries usually provide someone to meet the team and guide them through the official channels. At large events the immigration and customs officials will often provide special clearance channels for the teams.

Particularly when visiting unfamiliar countries the author's own practice is to make a point of declaring the medical supplies carried. So far, over a period of ten years, bags have not been searched. It is nevertheless a good idea to have a list of the contents available to show to customs officers if necessary.

Athletic events are usually held in towns rather than villages and one can usually rely on there being somewhere locally to obtain medical supplies. It may be a salutary lesson as to how much drugs actually cost. It may be helpful to carry some form of proof of identity and also of medical qualification. It is also useful to carry a *National Formulary* since the brand name of many drugs varies from country to country and the generic name may be easier to identify.

All major competitions require selected athletes to provide a specimen of urine for testing for banned substances. One of the functions of a team doctor is to accompany the athlete through the procedure. The doctor is not just there for moral support but also as an observer to ensure that the test is properly explained to the athlete and properly carried out. It is at this point that the doctor can make sure that any drugs and their dosage taken by the athlete for treatment are declared. In the event of a subsequent disagreement, and in some countries athletes found positive have disputed the matter in court, the doctor could be a material witness.

Conclusions and recommendations

The successful team doctor must have the capacity to come out from behind his or her desk, and be able to deal sympathetically

180

Chapter 12
Athletes at an
overseas venue:
the role of the
team doctor

with a collection of individuals, all of whom have extremely strong personalities and who are, in various ways, fired up to a considerable degree. The multiple roles of physician, surgeon, occupational health adviser, counsellor, dietician and masseur/masseuse are largely familiar to a family doctor.

Away from familiar surroundings it is harder to practise the same high standards of professionalism as at home, but maintenance of standards is, if anything, even more important away from home. The present equivocal status of sports medicine in this country, together with the peripatetic habits of athletes, has led to different ethical standards in terms of referral, either back to the GP or on to the specialist.

There is no question that high levels of physical activity lead to physiological changes and patterns of illness and injury that are unfamiliar in the general practice of medicine. Sports medicine is a speciality. It is to be hoped that its present struggles lead it to a mature status where it is recognised as a speciality in its own right and can fit into the conventional framework of medicine. Until then the present unsatisfactory state, where athletes' medical care is fragmentary, uncoordinated and, unfortunately, sometimes contradictory, will continue.

Medical records are a vital part of satisfactory care. It is difficult away from the convenience of secretaries and a regular orderly existence to exercise the necessary discipline to keep proper records, but this effort must be made.

It is perhaps time that some attempt was made by the sports governing bodies to set up a central system of record-keeping. A medical records clerk with computer aid could easily maintain a file to which access would be given to certain authorised doctors, which would include the athletes own GPs. A print-out for each athlete in the team would be given to the team doctor and returned to the central file with any new information.* Athletes would be encouraged to notify the governing body whenever they received treatment, perhaps by means of a personal log-book into which any treating doctor would make an entry and which would be reviewed by the medical record clerk at regular intervals. There is no reason why confidentiality should be sacrificed.

To be asked to be a team doctor is a privilege; it is also great fun. Away from your protective, and perhaps inhibiting, screen of receptionists, nurses and the general environment of surgery or clinic, you are accepted as a friend as much as a doctor. It is a friendship that can, in time, cover the world.

---

* Such a system might be of considerable benefit to individual athletes, but could only function with their informed consent. Subject to the provisions of the Data Protection Act, the information contained about an individual on computerised records would have to be available to that individual on demand.

Dental and facial damage in sport: risk management for general dental practitioners

13

R. W. KENDRICK

'What a word has escaped the barrier of thy teeth'
From the *Iliad* by Homer

Sports giving rise to dental and facial damage

Almost all sport can give rise to damage to teeth, mouth and face, though some sports, such as rugby, hockey, cricket and horse-riding, have been shown to be associated with a relatively high incidence of these injuries.

Dental or facial damage can occur due to contact with a club or stick, a ball, especially a hard ball, or another player's boot, fist or head. However, review of the literature would show that even such non-contact sports as tennis and walking have resulted in dental and facial injuries. In swimming, injuries result mostly from slipping on wet surfaces, but injuries due to diving or swimming into obstacles also occur. In horse-riding, particularly severe injuries are often seen, and these usually occur following falls from the horse or as a result of horse-kick injury. Cycling accidents can also lead to facial injuries, although most of these are not in the context of cycling as a sport.

Compton & Tubbs (1977) found that 7% (2128 patients) of patients attending the Birmingham Accident Hospital had injuries which had occurred during sport. La Cava in 1964, studying insurance claims for sporting injuries, found an annual average of 1.7% (8896 from 511 309) of those insured making a claim. Kramer in 1941 (quoted by Gelbier in 1966) found, in a study of 11 500 high school athletes enrolled in an Athletics Accident Benefit Plan, that there were 691 (6%) injuries requiring professional attention. Of these 159 were dental injuries. This represents 23% of those injuries and 1.43% of the total enrolled. Studies of the aetiology of maxillofacial injuries presenting to specialist units show that sporting injuries account for a range of 1.5% to 16.5% (Rowe & Williams 1985).

It should be recognised that there will be regional variations in the type of sport giving rise to injury. For example, Gaelic games are only played to any great extent in Ireland, and games such as bandy are native to the Soviet Union and Northern European countries.

181

182
Chapter 13
Dental and facial
damage in sport

A number of general principles can be considered in relation to prevention of dental and facial damage in all sports, and these will be discussed under the three main headings of interception, prevention and treatment.

Interception

It is important to recognise that, as well as, trauma, dental disease can affect a sports man's or woman's performance. Appropriate dental treatment may reduce problems in this regard and also the possibility of traumatic injury.

Interceptive treatment could really be considered as promoting general dental health and is not necessarily specifically related to sporting injuries. In relation to trauma, however, the special vulnerability of the incisor teeth needs to be considered. It has been shown in surveys that the correlation between the frequency and severity of fractures and the degree of protrusion of the incisor teeth is more than due to chance. Therefore, at the appropriate age, over-prominent incisor teeth are better corrected orthodontically to move these to a position where they are less likely to be traumatised, especially for those intending to continue participation in contact sport.

All players should be dentally fit. Team doctors and coaches should try to ensure that the players appreciate the need for this, especially just prior to a major competition or travelling to foreign countries. The loss of a player through being unfit due to dental problems, either from decay, apical abscess or infection around a troublesome wisdom tooth, is usually an avoidable problem. Severe dental pain often disturbs sleep despite treatment with large doses of analgesics, and this combination of pain and sleep deprivation will reduce the quality of performance or even prevent participation. Spreading dental infection or the removal of some wisdom teeth may require hospitalisation and the administration of a general anaesthetic, producing the need for a period of recovery. Wisdom teeth should not be removed during acute infection and therefore practitioners should make appropriate arrangements for sports men and women who have had a past history of dental sepsis. In this way treatment can be planned to minimise interference with training and competition schedules. The players should be made aware that it is impossible to obtain dental fitness through last-minute dental attention. Dental health requires ongoing and repeated attention to potential and established dental problems.

Prevention

The adage 'prevention is better than cure' may be profitably applied to dental and facial injuries. Prevention of such injuries should

183

*Chapter 13
Dental and facial
damage in sport*

ideally involve the governing bodies of the various sports, as well as individuals, parents, teachers and coaches.

It has been shown that the incidence of dental injuries is related not only to the type of sport but also to the age of the participant, the incidence decreasing with increasing age. It has been suggested that a learning process may be responsible for this trend, especially in certain sports such as horse-riding, swimming and golf. It is therefore important that adequate supervision is available, particularly for the beginner, where the combination of youthful enthusiasm and inexperience presents the greatest risk.

In the prevention of dental and facial injuries the use of mouth-guards and face-masks has been shown to be effective.

The mouth-guard, mouth-protector or gum-shield is appropriate equipment to be worn by all players participating in contact sports, and is compulsory in American football and boxing. However, to be effective, a mouth-guard must fulfil certain criteria:

1 It must fit accurately and should occlude evenly with the lower teeth and not 'prop' the occlusion.
2 It should have sufficient retention not to drop out during play, with the mouth open or as a result of a tackle.
3 It must be comfortable.
4 It must allow for normal breathing and as normal speech as possible.
5 It should cover the attached mucoperiosteum but not impinge on the soft tissue reflections of the mouth.
6 It must be made of a sufficiently resilient material to absorb the forces applied in both vertical and horizontal directions.
7 It must be large enough not to be inhaled or swallowed.
8 It must be easily made at an economic cost.
9 It should be capable of being kept clean and hygienic, with a surface texture acceptable to the wearer.

There are two main forms of the mouth-guard, either the proprietary, over-the-counter type, or custom-made.

Proprietary mouth-guards may be a simple channel of a moderately flexible plastic which corresponds to the outline of the average dental arch. One of this type may be softened in hot water and adapted to conform to the subject's teeth. These adapt relatively poorly, however, and are not recommended. Other proprietary mouth-guards are modified by infilling or loading the channel with a silicone material which adapts closely to the teeth and soft tissue while in its viscous state. This then 'cures' to provide a material which helps to absorb the shock of a blow and to stabilise the mouth-guard to an acceptable degree. These are, however, not suitable for markedly irregular or protruding teeth.

The custom-made mouth-guard requires the services of a dental surgeon and a dental technician, as it is made to models of the subject's mouth and teeth. It is usually made out of a heat-cured

184

Chapter 13
Dental and facial
damage in sport

silicone rubber or sheets of polyvinyl–polyethylene plastic which are vacuum-formed to models of the mouth and teeth. They are suitable for all cases and fulfil all the above criteria, but are, of necessity, more expensive than proprietary mouth-guards.

Individuals who are fitted with crown and bridge work, especially in the anterior part of the mouth, should be advised to wear a mouth-guard in contact sport. Players who have removable appliances should be instructed to remove these. A mouth-guard for these players should be constructed to cover the edentulous areas and the remaining teeth.

During orthodontic treatment a looser-fitting mouth-guard may have to be accepted so as to avoid prevention of planned tooth movements, and also to circumvent the need for frequent remakes of the mouth-guard.

Mouth-guards not only prevent dental damage but also help to reduce the incidence of soft tissue injuries and fractured jaws. Davies *et al.* (1977), in their survey, found that 45% of club rugby players had experienced a dental injury while playing, but none of these had been wearing a mouth-guard.

Mouth-guards also help to absorb some of the forces applied when the jaw is struck, especially when the clenched teeth position is adopted. This reduces the forces transmitted to the temporomandibular joints, skull and brain, and therefore helps to reduce the severity and incidence of acute and chronic brain damage.

In economic terms the value of a mouth-guard is well illustrated when it is realised that it costs approximately 5–10% of the cost of a porcelain crown for an anterior tooth.

Face-masks, if correctly designed and worn, are effective in preventing damage to the face and teeth, and, if extended to cover the skull, provide excellent protection for this area. However, they must fit accurately and be adequately retained. The helmet type of face-mask which incorporates facial and cranial coverage is preferable. The face-masks should not be solely supported on the facial bones as this type transmits the forces directly to the structures it is supposed to protect. Many goalkeepers in field- and ice-hockey have an additional extension to the helmet type of face-mask with a flap of padded material coming down from the mask to cover the otherwise unprotected throat and larynx. In sports such as cycling and horse-riding, helmets which include face or chin protection help to reduce dental and facial injuries and are recommended.

The Bureau of Dental Health Education of the American Dental Association estimated, in 1973, that, since the introduction of mandatory wearing of face-masks and mouth-guards for American footballers, 100 000 oral injuries had been prevented annually.

Governing bodies of sports have a responsibility for the prevention of accidents. They should advise or legislate within the rules of the game for players to be allowed to, or required to, wear ap-

185

*Chapter 13
Dental and facial
damage in sport*

propriate protective equipment. The example of American football illustrates dramatically the benefits to health which may accrue. Rules governing the type and condition of the sporting equipment used are important, and this would include such diverse items as sticks, helmets, goalposts, pitch surface and surrounds. It is the responsibility of the playing officials, referees, umpires and linesmen, etc. to check equipment before the players take the field. Match officials should order a removal of equipment that may have become dangerous through damage during play. Coaches and managers should be encouraged to ensure that players have maintained their sports equipment in a safe condition and that they make full use of protective equipment that is available.

Rules outlawing interpersonal violence are essential and must be strictly applied. Clearly this is an area which is and should be controlled by referees and disciplinary committees of the respective sports.

Treatment

While damage to the teeth, jaws and soft tissues may produce spectacular injuries, it must always be remembered that the general condition of the patient is of vital importance. Control of the airway, control of bleeding and assessment of the level of consciousness must still take priority, as with any accident victim.

Damage can occur to the hard tissues, i.e. teeth and bones, and to the soft tissues.

The extent of damage that occurs to the teeth from a direct blow can vary from no displacement of the tooth, to partial loss of tooth substance, to complete avulsion of the tooth from its socket. The tooth that has been traumatised with no loss of tooth substance can, however, suffer damage to its nerve and blood supply and may subsequently die. In cases where this has occurred the patient should be warned, and the vitality of the tooth monitored by the practitioner and appropriate radiographs taken when indicated. Root treatment and/or crowning may be required at a later date.

In young children, deciduous teeth which have been displaced usually require little treatment unless they are interfering with the bite or subsequently become infected. If the displaced teeth are interfering with the normal occlusion, then they need to be either repositioned or extracted. It is worth warning the parents that the permanent tooth may be displaced or damaged (dilacerated) by the trauma, but a 'wait and see' policy can only be adopted.

Damage to the permanent teeth should be actively treated. This treatment is based on Ellis's classification and a summary is shown in Table 13.1.

Fractures or displacement of the teeth may not always be obvious unless careful examination is undertaken. This is particularly so in

186

*Chapter 13
Dental and facial
damage in sport*

the vertically split tooth as seen in the premolar and molar regions, which may only be diagnosed with careful probing of the cusps of the teeth when acute pain will be produced. Fractured or displaced teeth may lead to a part or the whole of a tooth being embedded in the soft tissues of the lips or mouth, and therefore any laceration associated with damaged teeth should be carefully explored or X-rayed for this complication. Another rare complication is the inhalation or ingestion of a tooth or a tooth fragment. Should there be any suspicion that this has occurred, the appropriate chest and/or abdominal X-ray should be taken.

Damage to the soft tissues of the mouth and lips may or may not require suturing. The generous blood supply in this region means that healing is usually rapid and seldom complicated by infection. Minor abrasions or splits of the inside of the lips will often heal themselves without recourse to suturing. However, where the gingival margin has been displaced this should be accurately sewn back into position. In all cases of intraoral wounds instruction should be given with regard to oral hygiene to prevent secondary infection. Careful use of the toothbrush is mandatory, supplemented with hot saline mouthwashes or chlorhexidine mouth rinses as indicated.

Lacerations of the skin require careful cleaning and closure. A tattooed or stepped scar is very difficult to correct subsequently. Accurate suturing is especially important where the wound involves the vermilion border of the lip.

Damage to the bone of the jaw may involve the supporting alveolar bone of the teeth, in fractures of the jaw or cheek-bones. Fractures of the maxilla are relatively rare in sports injuries. Fractures of the cheek-bone and mandible, however, show a much higher incidence in contact sports. These may not be associated

Table 13.1 Treatment of damage to permanent teeth, based on Ellis's classification

Classification	Injury to tooth	Treatment notes
Class I	Enamel chipping only	Smooth enamel, ? composite restoration
Class II	Coronal fracture involving enamel and dentine only	Cover exposed dentine, e.g. Ca(OH)$_2$ ± temporary crown
Class III	Coronal fracture exposing pulp	If root has an open apex, carry out pulpotomy and cover with Ca(OH)$_2$ and zinc oxide/eugenol dressing. If apex closed extirpate pulp and root-fill
Class IV	Root fracture ± coronal fracture	Depends on the position of the fracture. Apical third fracture may require root extirpation ± splinting. Other fractures generally indicate extraction
Class V	Displaced tooth	If sufficient periodontal support, reinsert at the earliest opportunity and consider splinting, e.g. wiring or acid-etch to adjacent teeth. Minimum handling of root surface is important

Source: Poswillo *et al.* (1986), p. 13.

187

Chapter 13
Dental and facial
damage in sport

with displacement or marked symptoms, but their diagnosis is important as further trauma before healing is complete can lead to marked displacement and complications. It is therefore important following a blow to the face or teeth that the appropriate X-rays should be taken to exclude such fractures. This may even apply after a blow to a tooth with no apparent loss of tooth substance. This emphasises the point that it is important to make a thorough examination of the patient who has been injured.

Treatment follows the usual pattern of interdental and, where necessary, intermaxillary wiring for alveolar and mandibular fractures. Fractures of the middle third of the face (maxilla and zygoma) usually require referral to the appropriate hospital specialist.

It is usual to suggest a period of six weeks before recommencing playing after a simple zygomatic or mandibular fracture. In complex or comminuted fractures it may be necessary to advise the patient to avoid contact sports completely until solid clinical union has been obtained. This may be in excess of 12 weeks.

Conclusions and recommendations

Facial and dental damage can occur in almost all sports. The number and severity of these injuries can be reduced with the appropriate use of protective equipment and through legislators and officials framing and enforcing appropriate rules.

Patients who may be, or have been, involved in a sporting injury may present some legal pitfalls for the practitioner. These may arise from a failure to adequately warn or inform a patient of possible risks or complications, e.g. failure to warn a patient that a traumatised tooth may give rise to problems at a later date, or to advise a patient to wear a mouth-guard after crown and bridge work. Patients who wear removable appliances should be warned to take these out prior to participating in contact sports, or in situations where oral or facial damage is a possibility. Other problems may arise through failure to diagnose a split tooth, tooth fragments becoming embedded in the soft tissues, or an inhaled or ingested tooth. Failure to take appropriate X-rays may lead to an indefensible medico-legal position.

References

Compton B. & Tubbs N. (1977) A survey of sports injuries in Birmingham. *British Journal of Sports Medicine* **11**, 12–15.

Davies R. M., Bradley D., Hale R. W., Laird W. R. E. & Thomas P. D. (1977) The prevalence of dental injuries in rugby players and their attitude to mouthguard. *British Journal of Sports Medicine* **11**, 72–4.

Gelbier S. (1966) The use and construction of mouth and tooth protectors for contact sports. *British Dental Journal* **120**, 533–7.

188

*Chapter 13
Dental and facial
damage in sport*

La Cava G. (1964) The prevention of accidents caused by sport. *Journal of Sport Medicine and Physical Fitness* **4**, 221–8.

Poswillo D., Babajews A., Bailey M. & Foster M. (1986) *Dental, Oral and Maxillofacial Surgery.* London: William Heinemann Medical Books.

Rowe N. L. & Williams J. L. (eds) (1985) *Maxillofacial Injuries.* Edinburgh: Churchill Livingstone.

Vincent-Townend J. R. L. & Langdon J. G. (1985) Appendix. In *Maxillofacial Injuries,* vol. 2, ed. N. L. Rowe & J. L. Williams, pp. 999–1014. Edinburgh: Churchhill Livingstone.

Further reading

Blonstein J. L. & Cutler R. (1977) Mouth and jaw protection in contact sports. *British Journal of Sports Medicine* **11**, 75–7.

Hill C. M. & Mason D. A. (1985) Dental and facial injuries following sports accidents: a study of 130 patients. *British Journal of Oral and Maxillofacial Surgery* **23**, 268–74.

Jarvin S. (1980) On the causes of traumatic dental injuries with reference to sports accidents in a sample of Finnish children. *Acta Odontologica Scandinavica* **38**, 151–4.

Rontal E., Rontal M., Wilson K. & Barclay C. (1977) Facial injuries in hockey players. *Laryngoscope* **87**, 884–94.

Sane J. & Ylipaavalniemi P. (1987) Maxillofacial and dental soccer injuries in Finland. *British Journal of Oral and Maxillofacial Surgery* **25**, 383–90.